Law, Medicine, and Social Justice

Larry I. Palmer

Westminster/John Knox Press
Louisville, Kentucky

© 1989 Larry I. Palmer

Book design by Gene Harris

First edition

Published by Westminster/John Knox Press
Louisville, Kentucky

PRINTED IN THE UNITED STATES OF AMERICA

9 8 7 6 5 4 3 2 1

Library of Congress Cataloging-in-Publication Data

Palmer, Larry I., 1944–
  Law, medicine, and social justice.

  Bibliography: p.
  Includes index.
  1. Medical laws and legislation—United States.
2. Physicians—Malpractice—United States. 3. Medical
jurisprudence—United States. 4. Medical ethics—
United States. I. Title. [DNLM: 1. Ethics, Medical.
2. Jurisprudence. W 32.6 P174L]
KF3821.P35 1989   344.73′041   88-27936
ISBN 0-664-21333-2 347.30441

For
Barry, Isaac, and Reid

Contents

Acknowledgments

Three individuals deserve special mention for their assistance to me in this work. My colleague Davydd Greenwood encouraged me to write this book at a time when I was tempted to pursue only administrative concerns. He later chaired the steering committee of the Comparative Studies in Professionalism and Professional Education Program at Cornell, which offered me many opportunities to discuss the ideas presented here with colleagues from a wide range of disciplines. Collaboration with my colleague H. Richard Beresford of the Cornell Medical College, in teaching seminars and courses on law and medicine over the past ten years, provided the conceptual foundation. Roberta Armstrong carefully read the entire manuscript and gave critical advice in the final stages of the writing.

Many others have given support by reading and commenting on portions of the manuscript, among them Alexander Aleinikoff, Alfred Aman, Sander Gilman, Carol Greenhouse, Eugenia Hurme, Mary Katzenstein, Peter McClelland, Ruth Morse, and Sharon Rush. My students at the Cornell Law School and the Cornell Medical College, and the undergraduates in my Biology and Society courses in Cornell's Colleges of Arts and Sciences and Human Ecology, have also contributed greatly to the writing of this book. Patricia Lawrence, Jonathan Mintz, and Wendy Tarlow, students at the Cornell Law School, provided invaluable research assistance. I regret that the many others who helped with the book are too numerous to name.

I am grateful to former Deans Roger Cramton and Peter Martin of the Cornell Law School for making my collaboration with Dr. Beresford possible over the years and for providing both financial and logistical support. My work in the central administration at Cornell has never been a burden but has been stimulating to me, both personally and professionally. I am grateful to my colleagues who have provided such an exciting environment in which to work and for supporting my efforts to teach while I have served in administrative positions. When I left my first such position after five years, in 1984, the university generously provided me with a leave to begin this book. I am grateful to Sir Michael Stoker and the Fellows of Clare Hall, Cambridge University, for providing me with a congenial place in which to write a substantial portion of the first draft during the 1984–85 academic year. My thanks also to the Andrew W. Mellon Foundation, which, through its Fresh Combinations Programs, provided financial support for my work through Cornell's Program in Comparative Studies in Professionalism and Professional Education.

I also thank Keith Crim and Janet Baker of Westminster/John Knox Press for the care with which they handled this project, and Marcia Carlson for preparing the index.

L. I. P.

Ithaca, New York
January 1989

Introduction

The Search for Caring
and Justice

There is an underlying theme of hope in our present intense concern about the interaction between law and medicine. At the same time that we marvel at the tremendous achievements of modern medicine, we are faced with new moral dilemmas concerning health care. Surely our perplexities about law and medicine ought to be seen not as intractable conflicts between professionals but as a common search for caring and justice.

Posing the right questions is an essential feature of any social response to the moral and ethical dilemmas in law and medicine. We are not simply searching for better health care, or even a more humane medicine, but for ways to connect our present and ever-increasing technological capacity with those basic bonds that we believe hold human societies together—concepts of caring and justice. When our search for a new understanding for caring involves conflicts, we increasingly turn to law, not to find the right secular answer but to discover a new form of social harmony: a basic conception of justice.

When a legal conflict concerning medicine arises, it usually involves some allegation about a failure of care. Care should be broadly defined to encompass the whole range of a physician's role, from healer to technician, and the entire panoply of services provided by institutionalized medicine. As individuals who may become patients ourselves, most of us want more than technical competence when we are sick; we want the empathy of another human being, whether we suffer from a slight cold or terminal cancer. Although modern physicians are taught the scientific approach, our ideal physician remains the caring healer, who not only brings the insights of modern science to the patient's case but also alleviates the patient's suffering with emotional and perhaps even spiritual support.

When faced with conflicts involving the actual practice of medicine, we as laypersons want law to embody some notion of justice. For some, the concept of justice derives from ideals about law's obligation to protect individual liberty of action. Others may see justice as assuring equality of treatment. Still others judge legal decisions by whether the particular result helps enforce those values, such as respect for life, that are necessary for a just society in the long run.[1]

I question whether existing legal analyses can adequately resolve the underlying moral and social issues in medicine—or, for that matter, provide us with new ways of thinking about the social functions of medicine. Thus this book will examine current perspectives of law and medicine and propose that broad concepts of caring and justice serve as the best guides to judicial, legislative, administrative, and professional decision-making. In short, I shift the focus away from individual cases to the broader institutional functions of law and medicine. Modern medicine is more than individual professionals engaged in certain activities. It is a formal institution within society.

What are the forces shaping the institution of medicine today? We find, first, that the scientific orientation of medicine has an overriding influence on the behavior both of health care professionals and of potential patients. Second, the resulting growth of knowledge creates an impetus toward specialization among modern health care professionals. Third, a variety of organizations have come to comprise the institution, including hospitals, abortion clinics, mental hospitals, and health maintenance organizations. Fourth, third-party insurance, the primary method of financing health care in this country, helps to shape not only health care organizations but our ethical concepts about health care delivery as well.[2] The institution of medicine is thus a social construct that manifests itself in social and economic relationships within society.

Over the past forty years, developments in bioengineering, clinical pharmacology, and molecular biology have radically changed modern medicine and, consequently, the way health care is provided in the United States. The medical practitioner is heavily influenced by developments in the biomedical research laboratory. The modern scientific approach to medicine claims that the advancing technologies resulting from this research justify the taking of risks and the investment of resources and will eventually lead to greater social improvements in health and well-being. Ironically, with this advance in knowledge and technical capacity, we have become more aware of what is still unknown about medical intervention.

The public is increasingly uncomfortable with this "scientific ethos" of modern medicine. The most poignant manifestation of discomfort is the growing concern that medicine has now gained control over the process of death itself, thus eradicating the concept of "natural" death. Although most people no longer accept preservation of life at all costs as the goal of medicine, we are as yet unwilling to embrace an alternative that allows medical professionals to "dispense" death in certain cases. Abortion is another example of our public ambivalence about the role of modern medicine in our lives. While medical technology advances, we struggle to comprehend its implications and to make informed moral choices about its applications.

In the institutional approach taken by this book, law will be viewed as designed both to preserve the social order and to allow its evolution. Law is thus a social construct that depends on other social constructs—such as medicine and the family—for its social validity. Therefore the function of law in relationship to modern medicine must evolve, because the dynamic force of medicine is transforming our entire social order. At the same time, law also influences behavior (even when there is no active legal intervention), since it is an integral part of the way society and the its individual members perceive the social order. Moreover, legal professionals adjudicate disputes, promulgate rules and policies, and administer regulations in accordance with implicit and explicit concepts of how the social order is evolving.

Adopting an institutional perspective would change the role of legal intervention in health care decisions dramatically. Judges, lawyers, legislators, and administrative officials would first seek to understand the social and organizational context of the controversy before making any decisions regarding medicine. As legal decision-makers came to understand the larger social context, they would recognize that law's influence upon medicine as *practiced* is necessarily limited, but law's influence upon our *conception* of medicine's social role is potentially very great. Rather than seeking to regulate the individual doctor-patient relationship, law would aim to influence and direct the institutional structure of modern medicine. The ultimate goal of such an approach would be to increase the capacity of health care organizations, particularly hospitals, to regulate the doctor-patient relationship themselves. Law is, or should be, a last resort for maintaining the social order.

This institutional approach should not be confused with the increasing call for hospital ethics review committees or "institutional" review committees to advise or make recommendations to physicians and hospital administrators on the most difficult cases facing modern medicine. The proponents of such approaches do not realize that the very composition and powers of these committees are influenced by the social construct of modern medicine. Requiring that a committee review or advise does not necessarily provide a critical framework for assessing the influence of medicine on the social order. My approach requires that legal decision-makers make such assessments *before* devising a variety of processes to cope with the underlying social and moral conflicts.

The institutional approach builds upon some of the more profound scholarly critiques of law and medicine, which argue that the current reliance upon "informed consent" as the moral and ethical basis of legal decision-making in the medical arena is misplaced. There are two reasons underlying these criticisms.

First, granting to an individual the power to be a sole decision-maker in such situations as a severe physical or mental illness has destructive social and psychological consequences. When law delegates exclusive decision-making power to patients, their decisions lead to their psychological isolation. The perception of exclusive decision-making power is thus "anticommunal," because law is used to fracture the sense of social connections to the person most in need of societal care. To avoid these adverse consequences, law must acknowledge its own uncertainty when it intervenes in medical decisions and must therefore leave ultimate decision-making authority uncertain.[3]

A second problem is that the informed-consent approach does not address the fact that physicians traditionally rely on silence rather than dialogue in their contacts with patients. Many physicians do not share their doubts with patients in the face of the inherent uncertainty of modern medical intervention, because such sharing is seen as contrary to the physician's basic image of what it means to be a professional. To have true dialogue, both patient and professional must come to acknowledge these inherent uncertainties and learn to share the risks of treatment or no treatment.[4] Thus, the current reliance on informed consent masks assumptions about professionalism, expertise, patient knowledge, and patient capacity to understand, assumptions that need to be examined critically before being incorporated into legal doctrine.

Given this uncertainty within both law and medicine, I do not use existing biological concepts of "health" or "illness." Indeed, I take issue with the conventional view that health ought to be viewed primarily as a biological concept. A biological concept of health as either the absence of disease or the reconstruction of a fracture does fit well within modern medicine's belief that intervention is its primary task. Further, a biological definition of health might be useful to those wrestling with such intractable ethical or policy issues as "uncompensated health care" or "cost containment," because biological indices are more quantitative. But a biological definition does not deal with the underlying social concept of health that must be the foundation of any allocation of health resources, in accordance with social rather than individualistic images of justice.

In the institutional approach, there are two reasons why health must be seen as a relational or social concept. First, all societies have some general views about illness and death that relate to their basic beliefs about social interaction. Whether it be a clearly defined biological disease or a mental disease of uncertain origin, illness always represents a degree of social dysfunction. A social definition of health will help us understand, for instance, why societies with the same basic form of medicine and a legal system similar to ours (such as Canada and the United Kingdom) do not have the conflicts we have in this country over such issues as malpractice. The difference in legal treatment is, in my view, a function of the social organization of our respective health care delivery systems, not a function of a genetic defect in the American character that makes us more litigious than Canadians or the British.[5]

A second reason for using a relational concept of health is that it helps to overcome the assumption, implicit in most biological concepts, that health is a state which scientifically trained physicians dispense. A biological concept of health undermines the notion that individuals have the basic responsibility for self-care and discourages full discussion of the role of the prevention of illness in modern medicine.[6] A relational concept of health emphasizes the social context of doctor-patient transactions, including the fact that many patients do not share their physicians' view as to the best way to restore health or care for their illnesses.[7] A relational concept of health also helps us understand that many legal controversies are in fact disputes over the authority of individuals to take risks with their own lives or the lives of their children or wards.[8]

My goal in analyzing the interaction of law and medicine from the institutional perspective is to help us—layperson, physician, and lawyer alike—understand what we are trying to achieve through this interaction. We can then resist the growing tendency to use polemics in judging individual situations that are actually part of a larger context.

When an individual brings a malpractice suit or a hospital asks a court to determine whether the physician in charge of a case can terminate treatment, each comes before the court with a mixture of motives. But in all situations brought before law, broad social goals as well as the individual goals of participants must be considered. That is, for law to validate a litigant's personal motives, the litigant's goal must further some larger social goal that law has adopted. In this way we make each individual legal dispute a matter of public concern, thereby justifying the large social investment in the resolution of those disputes.

The search for these high ideals of caring and justice in individual disputes partially explains why there is so much conflict about values underlying the interaction of law and medicine. The concept of caring continues to evolve with successive biomedical advances. For some people, the entire concept of life and health has been challenged and questioned by the advent of test-tube babies. They long for a resolution that both recognizes the legitimate interests of others—those who desperately want children, for instance—and encompasses their personal idea of how best to respect "life." Since law is dependent on other social institutions for its evolving notion of the social order, it should come as no surprise that there is no consensus of what "justice" is in these increasingly numerous legal interactions with medicine.

The search for these ideals must be kept alive while we broaden our perspective to encompass the larger context in which these value conflicts are taking place. This perspective will help us devise ways to restructure the fiscal foundations of medicine, to reform the malpractice system, and to modify professional education.

Chapter 1

Liability Rules
and the
Entitlement to Health

Malpractice has become a battleground for physicians and patients, dominating most of law's relationship to medicine and allegedly driving up the overall economic and social costs of health care in the United States. The fear of lawsuits is believed to be the cause of "defensive medicine." It is the reason cited by some physicians who choose to forgo such specialties as obstetrics, where the cost of malpractice insurance is becoming prohibitive. It is also claimed that a small number of patients and the lawyers who represent them are beneficiaries of excessive monetary awards for relatively minor mistakes or unavoidable injuries.

Patients and their legal advocates counter with allegations that physicians have been given too much license. They contend that malpractice suits are a necessary corrective and allege that modern physicians are trained to treat only the disease, as opposed to considering the well-being of the "whole person." They argue that the possibility of a lawsuit protects the patient.

If, however, we were to use an institutional perspective and ask the protagonists in this struggle to define the term "malpractice," they would offer complex images of the way in which law and medicine should *not* interact. Almost all these images focus solely upon the doctor-patient relationship. For doctors, they often involve assertions that law, under the doctrine of informed consent, now requires them to give a litany of useless information to patients. Patients and their advocates, on the other hand, often view physicians as members of a self-protective guild that fails to police incompetence and often uses an authority derived from science to deceive patients through silence or misinformation.

We need to adopt an institutional approach to this complex system of legal rules called medical malpractice and focus on the functional definitions of legal rules, particularly liability rules.[1] Liability rules in medicine provide a degree of social protection that cannot be achieved easily or more cheaply by alternative means under our present organization of health care delivery. To do this, I will pose four questions about malpractice. They are summarized in the next four paragraphs, and then each will be discussed at length and illustrated.

First, how does law in U.S. society conceive of the "entitlement" to health? An entitlement is the first-order decision of any legal system about who will prevail between persons or groups with conflicting beliefs or interests. Since there is a great deal of conflict within our society about the meaning of health, it is important to have some understanding of how law, through a variety of legal rules, deals with health as a social concept. An analysis of the proposed sale of human body parts will illustrate how different kinds of legal rules—liability, contract, and criminal—operate together to help us understand law's definition of the entitlement to health. Unlike some scholars who might discuss "entitlements" to health *care,*[2] I analyze how law in our society conceives of the entitlement to health itself. Law as an institution does not provide health care; rather, law interacts with other institutions such as the family and medicine in helping to define society's concepts of health. From the perspective of law, the allocation and distribution of adequate food, exercise, medication, advice, and consulations from health care professionals—all of which are significant factors in individual and community health—are second-order decisions. The use of entitlement, in the sense of how law resolves a conflict, is not meant to denigrate the importance of these questions of allocation and distribution of health resources. Rather, the conflict definition of entitlement[3] is used to demonstrate that some entitlements are of such fundamental importance in our view of the social order that law will prohibit individuals from transferring the entitlement except through socially approved means. In the case of the entitlement to health, those socially approved means involve the institution of modern medicine.

Second, does society need liability rules in medicine at all? This question has surfaced in recent popular criticisms of the legal malpractice system. Judges have joined this debate by stating that the potential of malpractice suits inhibits physicians from making the correct ethical and moral decisions when confronted with inherently uncertain issues of modern medicine. This view was first expressed in the Karen Ann Quinlan case.[4] I would argue that the view expressed by the judges in that case was based on the prevailing simplistic approach to medical ethics in law. With an institutional view, on the other hand, the theoretical but seldom exercised right to bring a malpractice suit in a situation similar to Karen Ann Quinlan's is seen as an important and necessary part of the social control mechanisms we have devised for physicians and medical organizations.

Third, what is the nature of the social control function that liability rules would perform under an institutional approach? In addressing this question, I use this perspective to analyze a set of cases dealing with the responsibility of obstetricians to inform prospective parents of potential genetic defects in their offspring. This analysis demonstrates that such a perspective not only compels sensitive treatment of moral issues concerning the nature of life and emerging concepts of "genetic health," it also helps to create a better understanding of the transactions between patients and modern physicians within their institutional context.

Fourth, does the current approach to malpractice litigation, with its focus on issues of "informed consent," lead to the exclusion of medical organizations as potential social-control agents over medical professionals? Essentially, the current approach is a misdirected focus of law and has led to moral confusion, especially in the more highly sophisticated forms of medical intervention that can be characterized as experimental. An institutional approach shifts the focus away from the individual physician and onto the appropriate organization, particularly where innovative or experimental treatment is involved.

Viewing malpractice from the institutional perspective crystallizes the drawbacks of current approaches, which fail to consider the broader context of patient-physician transactions. The institutional approach considers medical malpractice as part of a liability system that is related to the manner in which society is organized and is developing. In particular, this approach assumes that the institution of medicine has a primary role in allocating and distributing health entitlements.

The Entitlement to Health

Jones, a man without a wife or children, places an advertisement in the local newspaper offering to sell his heart if and when needed for $50,000, payable now. Smith, a hard-working professional with a second wife, two children, and two stepchildren, is intrigued by the advertisement. With so much coverage of organ transplants in the news, Smith is aware of the scarcity of human organs for transplantation. He continues to smoke and drink heavily, even though his doctor reminds him every year that these activities increase the risk of heart disease. Smith wonders if he might purchase some "insurance" against heart disease by coming to an understanding with Jones.

Smith and Jones meet and work out an elaborate agreement that involves Jones's willingness to submit to a test for compatibility with Smith at a leading heart transplant center. Assuming a reasonable degree of compatibility exists, Smith is prepared to pay Jones $50,000 for a signed agreement that includes Smith's right to know of Jones's whereabouts at all times and to call upon him for his heart if the need should arise during Jones's lifetime. Smith also insists upon a performance bond from Jones that would pay him a large sum of money if Jones fails to voluntarily give up his heart when Smith "needs" it. Smith is willing to assume the risk of Jones's dying before he does, the attendant risks of keeping track of Jones, and the future risks of transplantation. The two men wonder whether the proposed agreement is enforceable as a legally binding contract.

We feel intuitively that their agreement is not legally enforceable because it offends some vague notion of justice. As legally trained persons we might assert that the purported contract is void because it is against "public policy": Jones might die in order for Smith to live. Obviously our legal system does not allow for contracts of homicide or, more important in the medical context, contracts of suicide. Even though Jones has been paid $50,000 today for his life sometime in the indefinite future, our instincts as laypersons would be to label a legal system that would enforce such a contract "unjust."

But if we ask what is unjust or exactly which public policy is violated, we begin to see the complexity of the situation. The loss of human life, for example, is not a deciding factor, since our legal system does allow for the sacrifice of lives to achieve such societal objectives as convenience or efficiency.[5] A little deeper probing into the allocation of human body organs for transplantation would make us even less certain of such an analysis. We know that the human organs available for transplantation are in short supply; not every patient medically certified as in need of a transplanted kidney, for instance, will receive one. We have recently undertaken a national effort to deal with this scarcity and to increase the supply.[6] I suggest that we first examine how we conceptualize the problem of shortages before we devise ways of allocating and distributing the organs that become available. We normally view this problem as an inability of the patients' medical caretakers to find an appropriate donor of the human organs. We seem to feel it is appropriate for someone to give a human organ but not to sell it to a particular person or to the highest bidder.

This analysis would make the Smith-Jones proposal appear, in theory at least, even more reasonable. Both Smith, the proposed buyer, and Jones, the proposed seller, have recognized something most of us refuse to see: health resources, including human organs for transplantation, are in very short supply. Under the circumstances, certain individuals might want to take political action to alter the current method of allocating human organs. Others, like Smith and Jones, might seek individual solutions to balance personal risk. Smith and Jones have simply decided to do something about the situation themselves. Smith, in effect, wants to buy private insurance against the need for a heart transplant, while Jones wants to capitalize on the uncertainty created by the scarcity of human organs for transplantation.

Despite the demonstrable logic and apparent reasoning behind the proposed Smith-Jones agreement, it remains at present a legal fantasy. While the law of contracts is an appropriate solution to many private needs, basic notions of the social order, rather than the failure to meet technical requirements for legal contracts, reject its use here. Although we accept organ donations as legal transfers, we are repelled by the suggestion of their sale. Slavery and prostitution are other examples of how society has come to reject the introduction of the human body into the "stream of commerce."[7] Even where there is an element of market commercialism in health transfers, medicine stills remains the mediator. This is especially clear in the sale of blood. Although the supervisory role of medicine is usually justified by the need to certify that the blood does not contain a disease such as the virus associated with Acquired Immune Deficiency Syndrome (AIDS), the system of medical certification allows institutionalized medicine to determine the social policies surrounding the transfer of blood in our society.[8]

We recognize that a person's health is partially a function of one's parents, one's environment, and other factors over which one has little or no control. But even if Jones could make himself or his family better off by the sale of his heart, law should refuse to recognize the agreement as a legally enforceable contract because most of us want to live in a society that treats human body parts as inalienable, not subject to private transfer. We implicitly fear the long-run effects upon society if law were to change and shape our attitudes to accept the selling of human body parts as a legitimate way of maintaining one's health.[9]

A further objection to the Smith-Jones proposal is based on our mistrust of the open market's ability to come up with the appropriate social allocations essential to such an important area as health. Our view of health within law is not based on using agreements between individuals as a means of allocating health, a social concept, although important group health insurance contracts do exist in health care delivery in the United States. But we feel it is morally ambiguous to decide which patients should have the available human organs. We usually devise social and political structures to avoid having any individual or group of individuals consciously choose one life over the other. In fact, these types of decisions—these "tragic choices"[10]—are usually made in a context that avoids a direct choice.

Our social response to the variety of issues associated with human organ transplantation has been to rely on regulation as opposed to adjudication of individual disputes. When kidney dialysis machines were first developed in the 1960s, hospital-appointed committees attempted to decide who should use them. These hospital-based committees' decisions were viewed as an illegitimate means of rationing the scarce health resource. Rather than develop a viable means of allocating this new medical technology, Congress responded in 1972 with a regulatory measure that provided federal insurance reimbursement for all renal dialysis—an attempt to increase the supply of machines and to avoid having to choose one patient over another. This federal legislation recognized the interrelationship between renal dialysis and the practice of transplantation and provided federal reimbursement for virtually all kidney transplantation.[11]

Even within this regulatory scheme of federal insurance reimbursement, two issues were left unresolved. First, even if we provide the fiscal support to pay for hospital personnel and the technology, how do we expect to obtain the kidneys for transplantation? Second, if there is a scarcity of kidneys, as surely we must have known there would be, how do we determine whose needs for a transplanted kidney will go unmet?

Our initial response in the kidney transplantation program was to rely on human compassion: a living donor with two healthy kidneys would give one to a patient in need of it. Early in the kidney transplantation program, the medical profession asserted that only persons related to the donor could be considered candidates for donation. The prevailing view of transplant specialists was that any stranger who wanted to give a kidney based on altruistic motives was probably psychologically disturbed. Only when the shortage of organs began to create more difficult moral situations for medicine and society were these objections displaced and steps taken to increase the supply. In particular, various state legislatures, actively supported by medical organizations, passed laws allowing people who die, particularly those who die accidentally, to donate their organs for transplantation.[12]

The mere passage of state laws permitting the donation of kidneys and other body parts did not provide enough organs to meet even the perceived need. An "anatomical gift," supposedly legally validated through signed donor cards, might not produce any organs if family members objected or if no one realized that the soon-to-be-declared-dead patient had in fact signed a donor card. Although in theory authorized to remove the organs, physicians generally were not prepared to act without consent from the donor's family or in the face of family objections.[13] Death is such a significantly taboo topic in this society that neither hospital personnel nor health care professionals seemed willing to inquire about whether there was a signed card for fear that they would be viewed as seeking the patient's death to help other patients.

Donation of human body parts upon death was soon seen not simply as a matter of two private individuals—one dead and one alive—arranging a gift. Rather, donation of organs requires a system or an organizational framework for bringing the donor (the Joneses of this world) and the recipient (the Smiths of this world) together in accordance with social norms rather than their own private values about health. This attempt to build a system—a form of community assessment of who should get the organs—will help us to see that we are still dependent on the institution of medicine as a means of achieving a fair and just system of allocating health resources. More importantly, we will see that our concept of health—what health means—is heavily dependent on heretofore implicit notions of medicine as an important social institution.

In 1984, Congress responded in a number of ways to the need to build a social mechanism for allocating resources devoted to organ transplantation. In addition to prohibiting the sale of organs, the National Organ Transplant Act of 1984 established a national organ-sharing system and established a multidisciplinary Task Force on Organ Transplantation to make recommendations on the whole range of issues associated with the procurement of human organs for transplant.

One result of these federal initiatives was the establishment of United Network for Organ Sharing by which a national system for allocating organs, supposedly more equitable and efficient, would be achieved. To build the national system, Congress used the incentive of federal reimbursement. That is, in order to receive federal reimbursement through Medicare and Medicaid, hospitals are required to be a member in the network. Under this system, patients are given ratings based on their medical urgency, length of time on the waiting list, and other factors. This information is available through a national computer network. In addition, when hospitals in the network obtain organs from cadavers, they must enter relevant information about the tissue into the network computer to allow for computerized matching. This system has all the appearances of "objectivity" and is the clearest recognition that we must ration and thus choose one individual as opposed to another to receive the scarce resource.

Having a method of allocation is not, however, a system for dealing with the social context of the medical practice of organ transplantation. Many steps must be taken if the system of national allocation is to be viewed as socially effective. In April 1986, after the task force had issued its recommendations and based in part on its findings, the Uniform Anatomical Gift Act was revised in an attempt to increase its efficiency as means of encouraging living persons to donate their organs upon death.[14] In addition, the task force recommended that a "Uniform Determination of Death Act" be enacted that would allow transplant teams to use "brain death" as a definition of death. Finally, the task force recommended that states enact statutes requiring hospital administrators to ask surviving relatives to donate organs when the decedent had *not* previously signed a donor card.[15]

There are many features of these new attempts to deal with organ procurement and allocation that are worthy of consideration, but my purpose in discussing transplantation is to help us see how we think about health in devising social schemes.

No system will meet all needs or solve all problems, and the new national system is already starting to create a set of new questions. Under this system of sharing organs, for example, a hospital may ship a kidney it might have otherwise used for one of its own patients to another hospital with a "better matched" recipient. While we might want to think that we have a national system that is objective in the sense that the selection process appears to done scientifically by computerized matching, we should recognize that health care officials still have the power to ignore the computerized match. Medicine, through its professionals, still remains the gatekeeper in the process of selection. It will also take some time for patients and their families to adjust to this system of living donation for kidneys and donation upon death for kidneys, hearts, livers, and other organs. The larger issue that remains to be solved is how do we develop a social concept of medicine that makes the discretion of health professionals, inevitable in any system, legitimate in the eyes of the community? It is apparent that our most recent attempts to deal with transfer of health from one individual to another is heavily dependent on donation upon death as the solution to scarcity. We have tacitly placed our faith in the social institution of modern medicine and its accompanying organization, the modern hospital, to make the fitting decision concerning the allocation of available human organs for transplantation.

Three features implied in the donation-upon-death solution to organ scarcity further center transplantation in the hospital. First, the donation upon death solution assumes that donors will implicitly accept new definitions of death instead of the traditional one based on the heart's stopping. These new definitions, relying in part on "brain death,"[16] have been developed in the last fifteen years as a partial response to the need for standards that clearly legitimate the practice of organ transplantation. Note, for instance, that a physician engaged in organ transplantation cannot declare the donor "dead" under the brain-death definition.[17]

Second, the place of donation is assumed to be a hospital because the procedure requires a surgical operation and correct medical handling of the organs in order to make them usable for transplantation. Furthermore, it is understood that medical personnel would execute the donor's intentions,[18] reassure the family of the moral correctness of the donor's decision, and generally exercise control at the point of death in the context of a modern hospital equipped to perform transplants.

And third, because transplants are hospital centered, it follows that we are relying on these hospital organizations to implement the social standards manifest in the numerous regulations and guidelines emerging from the state and national task forces on organ transplants.[19] It should be noted, for instance, that under the revised Uniform Anatomical Gift Act, the hospital, not the physician, is the legal recipient.[20] Federal regulations on reimbursement and on procurement of organs are directed at hospitals, even though their hoped-for or ultimate effect is on the behavior of health care professionals.[21]

While we recognize that no one person should make these fateful decisions, we are content to place our faith in modern medicine as an institution to make them. Without knowing precisely how the decision is made—for the most part we do not really want to know—we trust the hospital to decide "correctly." Yet even in this hospital-centered world, where a new concept of death based on modern medicine's needs has been introduced, the scarcity of human organs remains. The donation-upon-death solution has not, and from most points of view will not, eliminate the necessity of choosing one patient as opposed to another for the organ transplant.

In this complex world of modern medicine, it is possible to understand why Smith and Jones cannot make a transaction that involves a transfer of health from one individual to another. As a society, we have already made the decision that medicine, as an institution, will allocate and supervise transfers of health. If individuals view "health" differently, we leave it to medicine as an institution to resolve the possible conflicts. Law has validated this social decision by holding any attempts to negotiate transfers of human organs as void and unenforceable, thus having no legal effect. Law has gone even further and made the sale of human body parts a crime, reinforcing the notion that the entitlement to health is inalienable.[22] Therefore, it is the transfer of health entitlements by private agreement, not the threat to human life, to which law objects. We have little objection today to Jones's giving his heart to Smith under the correct (socially defined) circumstances, but the new version of the Uniform Anatomical Gift Act makes it clear that there can be no "commercial transaction" regarding the organs after the death of the donor.[23] The Smith-Jones agreement would still be void even if it were not life-threatening.

Since law has generally allowed medicine to be the allocator of transfers involving health, two questions in particular need to be addressed: What are the limitations on medicine? How do individuals complain about medicine's particular allocations and seek redress?

My hypothesis is that the system of liability rules—a mechanism by which after-the-fact law requires the payment of money by one party to another—is the major way in which law provides control over medicine's function as a transfer mechanism of health entitlements. Moreover, liability rules provide the means by which the health values of nonmedical persons are socially validated or invalidated. This liability system includes a host of legal doctrines built up by courts and legislatures under the rubric of medical malpractice.[24]

The Need for Liability Rules

Some physicians, along with their supporters among the judiciary, have argued that the more complex the ethical issues involved in a given case are, the more the uncertainty about legal results interferes with the appropriate social functioning of physicians in their transactions with patients. Under such an analysis, physicians would be entitled to more precise liability rules and, in certain cases, to total exemption from even potential liability. This claim was most forcefully set forth by the judges who decided the case of Karen Ann Quinlan.

In re Quinlan[25] posed the question of whether Karen Ann's father, as her guardian, should be permitted to order her physicians to remove the respirator believed to be sustaining her life. In a long opinion, the court held that the father could order her physicians to remove the respirator under certain specified conditions and that, if the physicians followed those procedures, they would be exempt from potential civil and criminal liability. Seen from the institutional perspective, this decision was based on a misunderstanding of the purpose of liability rules in shaping our attitudes and beliefs about health.

The trial court in *Quinlan* concerned itself with the physicians' reasons for not complying with the father's request to remove the respirator without judicial intervention. In that court's view, Karen Ann's physicians were acting in accordance with prevailing medical standards, since Karen Ann was, by any medical standard, alive (although unable to communicate because of a deep and persistent coma). In other words, physicians do not remove life-support systems from patients who are by definition alive. The court stated that the physician is "to exercise in the treatment of his patient the degree of care, knowledge, and skill ordinarily possessed and exercised in similar situations by the average member of the profession practicing in the field."[26]

Although the court did not acknowledge this directly, its statement of the physician's duty is taken from court-developed rules on liability for malpractice. The lower court reasoned that the physicians might be civilly liable for removing the respirator, since such an action would not be in accordance with "existing medical standards and practices," as defined by law. Thus the standards for the medical profession, in light of the moral ambiguity of Karen Ann's case, were initially enforced by succumbing to the gravitational pull of liability rules.

The appellate court reasoned that existing medical malpractice standards had prevented the lower court judge from authorizing the removal of the respirator. The court was cognizant that the Quinlan case was not a medical malpractice suit or, in my terms, a suit about liability rules. It was, in fact, an action for "declaratory relief," aimed at delineating the legal rights of the physicians and the guardian.

Moreover, the court proposed to assess the impact of the potential malpractice liability in the light of new medical technology sustaining Karen Ann. The court stated:

> The modern proliferation of substantial malpractice litigation and the less frequent but even more unnerving possibility of criminal sanctions would seem, for it is beyond human nature to suppose otherwise, to have some bearing on the [medical] practice and standards as they exist. The brooding presence of such possible liability, it was testified here, had no part in the decision of the treating physicians. . . . [W]e afford this testimony full credence. But we cannot believe that the stated factor was not a strong influence on the standards, as the literature on the subject plainly reveals.[27]

The court went on to note that the medical standards derived from general liability rules were ambiguous when applied to such problems as those presented by Karen Ann Quinlan.

Thus, in the appellate court's view, some type of immunity from potential civil and criminal liability was needed in order to "free physicians, in the pursuit of their healing vocation, from possible contamination by self-interest or self-protection concerns which would inhibit their independent medical judgments for the well-being of their dying patients."[28] The court sought to enhance the cultural ideal of the physician as healer by removing the inhibitory potential of liability in this difficult case.

But the opinion fails to note that death in the medical context is part of a larger concept—health. Liability rules are concerned with distribution of the more inconclusive notion of health values. Liability rules are not concerned directly with our attitudes about death except to the degree that those rules seek to encourage or discourage certain behavior or certain attitudes toward death on the part of physicians.

It is important to remember that liability rules come after the fact, when a result that a person views as adverse or somehow "bad" occurs. In contrast, the suit in *Quinlan* was an attempt to formulate a legal judgment *before* any course of action had been taken by the parties. Let me illustrate this point by using a hypothetical situation. Suppose that the physicians had removed the respirator when Karen Ann's father first made his request and that she had in fact died quickly. Suppose the father then brought a lawsuit against the physicians claiming that they had failed to inform him of all the pertinent medical facts before removing the life-support system, to wit: Karen Ann was not dead by medical standards and her case was medically unique (no one of her age had remained in a persistent coma for such a long time). Furthermore, in order to have any chance of success, her father would have to state that he would not have ordered the respirator removed had he been informed of these additional facts.

This hypothetical situation does contain a number of realistic uncertainties that would make the removal of the respirator risky, engendering a certain amount of caution on the part of Karen Ann's attending doctors. But this cautious attitude is precisely what we want in physicians. Since the removal of the respirator would involve the possibility of the patient's death, law should adopt a posture that encourages physicians to be cautious.[29]

When we consider some other facts of Karen Ann's actual case, it is perhaps easier to understand why the physicians forced the father to go to court. Despite his testimony in court, we should remember that he was ambivalent for a long time and had, in fact, given the physicians contradictory instructions.[30] In addition, there was some evidence by the time the case went to trial that Karen Ann could survive if she were gradually weaned from the respirator, although there was no evidence that she would ever recover consciousness.

The irony in this case is that Karen Ann Quinlan did survive the removal of the respirator and continued to "live" in a nursing home for eight more years; she died in June 1985. There are still many moral and ethical uncertainties and medical mysteries surrounding her case, but I maintain that the uncertainty of the law of medical malpractice contributed in a positive way—it made the physicians cautious. Had they been sure there would be no potential personal legal liability, they could have reacted to the father's natural ambivalence and chosen a premature death by removing the respirator. The uncertainty also encouraged a group consensus, even though it was not arrived at in this particular case. In the normal course of events, we would not expect the parties to go to court but to take the time to arrive at a decision to which all agreed. This group process would recognize the validity of a father's ambivalence about authorizing steps that would lead to his daughter's death.

Legal immunity for the physician, on the other hand, would allow the imposition of his or her own view of health on the situation, since there would be no outside corrective device for reviewing the physician's decisions. Certain individuals in our society, including some physicians, might feel that Karen Ann's health would have been better served if the respirator had been removed earlier and she had died. The entire court opinion, for instance, assumes that Karen Ann will die immediately if removed from the respirator and that certain death would be less painful than her supposedly intolerable position.[31] Rather than simply allowing a patient to die, such a view comes very close to a deliberate taking of life. Law should do as much as possible to neutralize the power of such views.

The court's ruling on immunity from liability included immunity from criminal prosecution. That the court chose to link the two forms of legal intervention—civil and criminal—points to a problem in liability rules not discussed in the court's opinion. The finding of civil liability against a physician implies that he or she has failed to meet the standards of the medical profession and is in some way "at fault." Criminal liability further carries the connotation of fault of a much more serious nature. If physicians were criminally responsible to society for their conduct (in the Quinlan case; for murder or manslaughter by removing the respirator too soon),[32] it is usually assumed that they would also be civilly liable to the plaintiff's estate. Thus there is a relationship between liability rules and criminal sanctions, but there is an enormous difference between the functions of both kinds of legal rules that the court does not take into account.

If we were to examine the Karen Ann Quinlan situation in terms of contract rules, we would be concerned with what Karen Ann and her physician had agreed to before she became a patient. Since she became a patient while unconscious in an emergency, the court would posit that a contract existed between the two parties. However, such an implied contract is not valid, as health is not a quantifiable commodity and, as such, is unsuited to the contract model. Parties' risks, expectations, and moral uncertainty are too extreme; they cannot legitimately contractualize away these difficult issues. Thus the contract cannot be just or morally acceptable. We have chosen instead to use liability rules. In liability rules the evaluation of allegedly impaired health is made socially or objectively: that is, by having a jury determine the legal effect of the negotiations and the extent of the injury to health. Under a liability rule, before determining injury value, a jury would want to look first at the physician's assessment and then at the patient's own assessment of the health values.

Criminal regulations are invoked when society has decided that certain fundamental rules about relationships between persons have broken down. If, contrary to prevailing medical standards, a physician removes a respirator, that physician may be liable to pay compensation if a judge and jury find malpractice. On the other hand, he or she would not be criminally liable unless there were a "clear social duty" not to remove the respirator. In the Karen Ann Quinlan situation, the possibility of criminal sanctions seemed remote indeed, much more remote than malpractice liability.

In specialized fields of medicine in which modern biomedical techniques are readily available, a physician can all too easily become the "dispenser of death" rather than the traditional "preserver of life." Liability rules provide the necessary check to professional behavior and thus provide a positive social good. The only reason put forth by the *Quinlan* court for exempting physicians from liability was its assertion that the potential of liability encourages physicians to act in terms of their own self-interest rather than the patient's interests.

To remove the potential of liability would allow a physician's self-interest, including the physician's own particular view of health, to predominate in doctor-patient transactions where death is a distinct possibility. (The Quinlan case is more than a question of somatic illness; her case has implications for how we deal with incurably ill mental patients who are by all accounts socially dysfunctional.) Thus, the more complex the medical and moral situation, the more we need the potential of law to intervene in the form of liability rules.

Judicial Attempts to Define Liability Rules

Although we have begun to rely on regulation rather than adjudication to resolve many of the basic issues facing law and medicine, courts play an important role in this society in defining law as an institution. Much of the legislation that seeks to resolve a great moral dilemma of our times, such as the appropriateness of "surrogate parenthood," is responsive to judicial attempts to resolve those issues.[33] It is thus important to see how judges could respond more effectively to a call for an institutional approach to law and medicine. Also it is important for nonlawyers to understand the kind of "generative metaphors"[34] that judges and lawyers use as they resolve important policy issues in the course of adjudication.

Judicial attempts to determine if physicians should be liable for failure to provide information about possible genetic anomalies in a fetus provide an example of how liability rules could operate in the morally sensitive area of genetic health. There are several features of these cases to bear in mind as we consider situations where the only therapeutic alternative is abortion. First, the physicians involved are specialists, and the liability rules developed in the cases ought to apply only to specialists in obstetrics as opposed to the more general class of physicians. Second, the practice of placing oneself under the care of an obstetrician rather than a general practitioner during pregnancy is widespread in America.

If pregnancy itself is not classified as a medical disease, we might ask ourselves: What is the purpose of consulting an obstetrician, a highly trained specialist in the delivery of babies? In any event, we should characterize the transaction between the obstetrician and patient as one involving a transfer of health values. The obstetrician fulfills a duty initially by constantly monitoring his or her patients— the mother and child to be—which at the primary level involves office visits and clinical tests.

The *Howard* v. *Lecher*[35] case offers a concrete example of this transaction and the attendant liability claims. In 1972, the Howard baby was born with Tay-Sachs disease, which affects the central nervous system, and within two years the child died. The parents brought a lawsuit against the obstetrician, Dr. Lecher, seeking to recover damages for the emotional and mental pain caused by seeing their daughter suffer and eventually die. By the 1970s, it was already widely known in medical circles that Tay-Sachs disease was caused by a genetic disorder. The incidence of the disease in the United States is 1 in every 360,000 births, but when both parents are of Eastern European Jewish backgrounds, it rises dramatically to 1 in every 3,600 births. At the time, clinical tests for Tay-Sachs were available; a simple blood test could determine whether the parents were carriers of the gene for Tay-Sachs, while another test, amniocentesis, could determine if the fetus had the disease.

Therefore, the Howards based their malpractice suit on the theory that Dr. Lecher, as part of his role as obstetrician, should have investigated the genetic history of the couple. Had he done so, Dr. Lecher would have discovered that both Mr. and Mrs. Howard were of Eastern European Jewish ancestry and were at greater risk of having a baby born with Tay-Sachs. The Howards further asserted that had they been informed of the availability of the tests, they would have undergone them and, upon discovery of the disease, would have aborted the fetus.

Dr. Lecher, however, took the position that he was not legally responsible for the emotional and mental anguish suffered by the Howards. He put forth a number of theories to support his position; the courts accepted the one that held that law should not compensate individuals for emotional injury when it did not accompany personal physical injury. In other words, American law recognizes that physical injury often entails some emotional suffering as well, and that it is both the physical and the emotional pain that entitles the injured party to compensation. This proposed lawsuit was outside the limits of these particular liability rules because the Howards themselves were not physically injured. Lawyers would say that Dr. Lecher was being sued for "mere emotional injury."

The New York courts, however, were not able to sweep away the emerging issues concerning the law's response to medicine's increasing knowledge about genetic defects. Only a year after the *Howard* v. *Lecher* case, the court was faced with another suit that raised similar issues of alleged physician malpractice.

Mrs. Becker, a woman of thirty-seven, gave birth to an infant with Down's syndrome. During the greater part of her pregnancy, Mrs. Becker was under the care of Dr. Schwartz, a specialist in obstetrics and gynecology. She and her husband brought a suit against Dr. Schwartz on the theory that he never advised Mrs. Becker either of the increased risk of Down's syndrome in children born to women over thirty-five or of the availability of amniocentesis to determine whether the fetus she was carrying had Down's syndrome. Like Mrs. Howard, Mrs. Becker contended that, had the obstetrician made her aware of the facts as well as the availability of the tests, she would have elected to abort the pregnancy once the chromosomal condition had been detected. In addition, the Beckers added several new dimensions to the courts' discussion of the implications of new developments in genetics on law, since they brought the lawsuit not only on their own behalf but also on behalf of their child. The court held that the mentally retarded child could not recover anything from Dr. Schwartz, reasoning that in this case awarding any compensation would imply that an infant has the "right" to be born "healthy."[36]

The court, however, held that the parents could recover from Dr. Schwartz the amount of money they would have to spend to care for their mentally defective child in an institution—the amount of extra expense associated with having a severely mentally retarded child as opposed to a child without such impairment. The exact formula for determining the damages was left to subsequent adjudication. On the other hand, to be consistent with *Howard* v. *Lecher,* the court held that the parents could not recover damages for any emotional injury or psychic distress allegedly caused by the birth of a Down's syndrome child.[37]

The New York courts have developed a doctrine of liability rules which holds that where knowledge about genetic defects is widely known among specialists in obstetrics, a physician is legally obligated to share that knowledge with the patient. Failure to do so could leave the obstetrician liable to the parents for expenses associated with caring for the handicapped child.

The New Jersey courts, faced with similar issues, held differently. In the case of *Berman* v. *Allan,* under circumstances comparable to *Becker* v. *Schwartz,* the New Jersey Supreme Court held that the parents of a child with Down's syndrome could recover for emotional distress caused by the birth of their mentally retarded child, but not for the amount of money spent in its special upbringing.[38] Like the New York courts, the New Jersey court held that the child could not recover anything for being born mentally impaired.

There are two differences between the ways the New Jersey and the New York courts interpreted the issues of sharing and using genetic knowledge. The first is that the two state courts began their respective analyses of the problem at different points. The New York court adopted a line of reasoning based on the public policy implications of a legal requirement to transfer money for "mere emotional distress." This line of reasoning ignores one of the fundamental tenets of liability rules, which requires an assessment of the duty imputed to a particular party to act in a certain way. In terms of entitlements, the New York court had to decide whether law should recognize the entitlement to certain knowledge about genetic health. Given the posture of the case in *Howard* v. *Lecher,* the court assumed that although Dr. Lecher had breached his duty by not in-

forming Mrs. Howard of the risks of Tay-Sachs disease, the issue of
damages for emotional injury was sufficiently overriding that they
could sidestep the analysis of the possible duty to inform the patient.[39]

In contrast, the New Jersey court started its analysis by considering a previous case dealing with similar issues,[40] specifically rejecting
the line of reasoning dependent on the question of whether damages
were too speculative. Instead, the New Jersey court focused its attention on the question of whether law ought to recognize a duty on the
part of the physician. As to the parents' claim, the court specifically
held that the obstetrician had deprived the mother of the right to at
least make a meaningful choice about continuing the pregnancy.
However, the court held that the child could not recover anything
because, in the court's view, the claim was based on the unacceptable
assumption that nonlife was preferable to life of a certain quality.[41]
An analysis of the question of "duty" in liability rules, as in the New
Jersey approach, allows the court to ask a host of questions about
the doctor-patient relationship in the context of modern medicine
that are masked under New York's broad statements about "public
policy."

The second major difference involves the implications of legalized
abortion. How can the knowledge of prenatal genetic disorders be
integrated into liability rules? In *Howard* v. *Lecher,* the judge writing
for the majority of the court made no mention of the availability of
abortion in connection with his public policy discussion. Abortion
was not part of the public policy debate, even though the dissenting
judge based his entire opinion on the availability of legal abortions
in the United States.[42] Only in its subsequent opinions in *Becker* v.
Schwartz did the New York court integrate the right of abortion
when it held that parents could recover for "pecuniary loss." The
New Jersey court, on the other hand, treated the availability of legal
abortion as the prime reason for overruling its previous decision,
viewing abortion as a therapeutic alternative to giving birth to a
defective child. Citing the constitutional right to an abortion, the
New Jersey court reasoned that the liability rules must be changed
accordingly. It felt that the public policy debate must now include
the fact that women have a legal right or an entitlement to abortion.

By starting with an analysis of the implications of the highly
emotive issue of abortion, the New Jersey courts conceived of the
entitlement to health in terms of the patient's need to obtain some
form of assistance from the physician. Since such an entitlement
exists, the court reasoned that the physician could have in fact damaged the patient emotionally and psychologically by failing to investigate the genetic background of the parents. The New York court,

by looking at the result of an impaired child as the measure of damages, implied that the patient's entitlement is constrained by the physician's need not to be subject to damages that are too "speculative." In contrast to the difficulty of setting a figure for emotional injury, the amount of money needed for medical care and rehabilitation of the child is fairly easy to estimate.

Since the New Jersey court focused on the emotional distress of the parents as the basis of physician liability, the duty imposed upon the physician may in fact be more uncertain from the physician's point of view than in the New York rule. In more practical terms, the physician's insurance company can ascertain the financial risks involved with medical expenses for children born with certain defects but would have great difficulty in determining the way in which a jury might value the emotional distress of the parents under the New Jersey rule.

As we evaluate the two different rules and their effects, one might feel that the New York doctrine is preferable because it provides greater certainty to physicians and their insurers about the potential costs associated with being a physician. One might also argue that we all benefit from more certain rules, since they allow us to purchase health services in a system where costs can be properly estimated. Whatever the benefits of certainty in other areas of law, however, the New Jersey rule, with all of its attendant uncertainty, has the more appropriate understanding of the purposes of liability rules in doctor-patient transactions concerning the sharing of genetic knowledge.

Given the monitoring function of the obstetrician, we must first decide the means of making the growing body of knowledge about genetic disorders socially useful, given that often the only medical alternative to an impaired child is abortion—which remains, at the very least, socially controversial. The law, as opposed to other institutions such as the church, ought to look first to existing legal precepts in deciding whether or not it will impose the view that abortion is a therapeutic alternative. The U.S. Supreme Court has already indicated in a series of opinions that a woman has a constitutional right to make the choice about whether or not to have an abortion. In fact, the Court early on restricted not only the legislatures' ability to deny access to abortion but also the power of hospitals and medical professional organizations to restrict a woman who has found a physician willing to perform an abortion from having one.[43] Thus, regardless of the physician's personal view or even the views of the community at large about abortion, genetic knowledge cannot legally be withheld from the patient.

Second, we must decide which of the two parties—the obstetrician or the patient—should have the responsibility for determining the potential for genetic defects. Since genetic disorders are predicated on genealogy, we could decide that the patient has the primary obligation to investigate his or her genetic makeup. Under such a view, any person contemplating having children should see a genetic counselor, a specialist who need not be a physician. On the other hand, we could determine that the obstetrician, as a medical specialist having greater access to the growing knowledge about techniques for detecting genetic abnormalities, should have the primary responsibility for raising the issue or, at the very least, should know enough to refer those patients who might be at risk to genetic counselors.

If we emphasize that the physician is a specialist rather than a general practitioner, this latter view would seem the more reasonable. In determining that the obstetrician is liable for the growing body of knowledge about genetic defects, law implies such knowledge must be shared with the patient in the course of periodic monitoring.[44] In this view the issue is not whether the baby is "normal" but whether the patient's sense of "health" and thus her values about health are allowed to enter the transaction. The most effective way to ensure that the patient's views of health would be meaningful in a doctor-patient transaction is for law to provide a framework for dealing with the emotional and moral issues at stake, while allowing for a degree of uncertainty.

The uncertainty of the New Jersey rule regarding potential damages for the emotional distress of the parents has the advantage of structuring the doctor-patient transaction in a socially useful manner. In scientifically oriented medicine, it is all too easy for physicians to calculate the value of their services in economic terms—the costs, for instance, of caring for a mentally retarded child—for these are "objective." A legal analysis that focuses on the potential emotional damage encourages obstetricians to individualize their practice—to engage in a form of caring. By so doing, law increases (but does not guarantee) the opportunities for the patient to discuss her attitudes toward health with the physician. This analysis encourages the obstetrician to treat the patient's view about the unborn child as important as his or her own scientific and personal views about children.

The New Jersey rule highlights the uncertainty of the effects upon the parents of having an impaired child or a child who dies shortly after birth. One reason for this uncertainty is simply the novelty of the legal issues involved. Lawyers have not had much experience with jury reaction to cases involving physicians' failure to warn of possible genetic defects in the unborn child.

The concurring justice in the New Jersey court would have taken the majority's opinion even further. He reasoned that the physician's failure to inform Mrs. Berman of the risks of Down's syndrome not only caused her emotional distress, by depriving her of her choice, but also led to an impairment of her and her husband's "parental capacity." The justice wrote:

> A full perception of the mental, emotional—and, I add, moral— suffering of parents in this situation reveals another aspect of their loss. Mental, emotional and moral suffering can involve diminished parental capacity. Such incapacity of the mother and father qua parents is brought about by the wrongful denial of a reasonable opportunity to learn of and anticipate the birth of a child with permanent defects, and to prepare for the heavy obligations entailed in rearing so unfortunate an individual.[45]

Furthermore, the justice reasoned that the child did have a legal basis on which damages could be recovered. Rather than characterize the child's lawsuit as a claim of "wrongful life," the justice structured the child's lawsuit as deriving from the physician's primary duty to the parents.[46] Under this formulation the child would be seeking damages for the mental and emotional harm of having been born to parents with an impaired parental capacity.

An immediate objection to the concurring justice's proposed rule would be the difficulty in separating the emotional harm to the parents from the emotional harm to the child. Under such circumstances, the physician might be forced to pay twice for the same breach of legal duty. This traditional objection to recovery could be overcome by subsequent refinement of the damage rules should a court be convinced, as a matter of policy, that the additional uncertain threat of the child's lawsuit would promote better treatment of the issues of genetic health.

With a degree of uncertainty in the liability rule, however, the child's lawsuit would be unnecessary. Rather than focusing on compensating past injuries, the more important function of liability rules would be to encourage or discourage certain conduct. In this way the liability rule performs the function of deterrence.

When dealing with deterrence within law, however, sanctions encourage some individuals to react in the desired way and at the same time encourage others to react in an undesired way.[47] The child's lawsuit is rejected in partial recognition that liability rules could lead physicians to engage in what has been called "defensive medicine," a generally undesirable practice.[48] However, there is no conclusive proof that new legal rules are the sole cause of physicians practicing defensively. Furthermore, present liability rules have not been explained to physicians or to the public in terms that emphasize the social function of the physician in relation to the growth of genetic knowledge. Rather, the rules have been interpreted in terms of the individual fault of the physician without consideration of the social context in which he or she operates. Within the function of liability rules suggested here, society, rather than the profession, has the opportunity to condemn the conduct of individual professionals as being below desirable standards.

Liability Rules in an Institutional Approach

When analyzing the decision-making authority of a patient in a medical transaction, American law looks to the ideal of the patient as a free and autonomous individual. The oft-quoted words from an early case discussing physician liability epitomize this ideal: "Every human being of adult years and sound mind has a right to determine what shall be done with his own body."[49] Modern law attempts to implement this ideal in doctor-patient transactions by basing physician liability on "lack of informed consent."

By most serious accounts, present legal attempts to supervise the doctor-patient transaction fail to obtain the ideal of the patient as a free, autonomous decision-maker. Rather than present refinements of this legal doctrine, I propose an alternative model of joint decision-making, which encourages true communication between physician and patient. This model confronts the problems of authority, autonomy, and uncertainty by imposing an ethical obligation on physicians to converse with patients about the inherent uncertainty of medical intervention. Through these conversations, patients come closer to the ideal of the autonomous individual within doctor-patient transactions.[50]

The prevailing joint decision-making model is flawed because it accepts that law's goal should be to make the patient a free and autonomous decision-maker. If the patient actually becomes a free decision-maker, we would conceptualize his or her relationship to the physician as a type of contract, allowing for the inequality of expertise. Although the contractual model is useful in comparison to the informed consent doctrine, it takes the autonomy of the patient too far. Society does not accept contractual transactions involving health. Although law may view the delivery of health care as a contract, law rejects the use of market forces, which are the underpinnings in the contract model, in structuring the overall doctor-patient relationship.

There are two dangers inherent in the contractual approach to medical ethics. First, the contract ideal encourages both a minimalist and a maximalist approach to the patient. Under a contract ideal, the physician will do only that which is required by the particular agreement; on the other hand, a contract notion of ethics encourages overkill in the form of defensive medicine in a world of increasing physician liability for malpractice. Second, the contract ideal encourages individuals to concentrate solely on their self-interests in matters of health. The problem here rests in the precariousness of each person's ability to direct his or her own health care.

There are, of course, other models for the doctor-patient relationship on which distribution of decision-making authority between physicians and patients might be based.[51] We seek an image as well as a concept that accommodates the themes of both justice and caring. We can find such a concept by seeing the modern physician and the patient as morally and socially bonded through their commitment to health. Under this view, health is not simply a biological state but a mutual goal, to be achieved through efforts on the part of both physician and patient.

When the patient and the physician are mutual partners in preserving health, the concept of disease changes from an extraordinary event that the doctor expertly manages to a process in which the patient and the physician both have a role. Physicians' professional commitment to health would mean monitoring the health of patients increasingly under the mutual partners model rather than under the contractual model. Physicians would seek to maintain health through preventive medicine rather than by expending most of their energies on the cure of illness.

Second, accountability to patients becomes a social matter instead of remaining simply a question of whether an individual physician did a proper job. The notion of a partnership in preserving health reminds the physician to look beyond the individual patient in thinking about his or her professional role. It encourages the medical profession to ensure that the whole of medicine—the hospital, the clinic, the research laboratory, and the professional organizations— are accountable to the public.

Third, the ideal of mutual health partners helps us to reflect on the specific doctor-patient relationship, as well as medicine in general, in terms of larger social obligations. In other words, we begin to set limits on the social value of health in light of other priorities. We could develop an analysis to combat the emotive quality of "No price is too high to pay for human life or good health" and yet have a socially compassionate system of medical ethics. Such a changed perspective would have greater significance as more and more of our gross national wealth is spent on health care.[52]

Not surprisingly, with various discussions of the underlying models of the doctor-patient relationship, American courts moved to modify liability rules in the 1970s. The theory of informed-consent liability discussed at the beginning of this chapter has gone beyond that of most other common law jurisdictions:[53] a physician is now potentially liable if he or she fails to inform patients of the inherent risks of a medical procedure.[54] Such a liberal rule simply formalizes the interaction between physicians and patients in highly specialized forms of medicine.[55] The courts have not, however, gone beyond the doctrine of informed consent and encouraged hospitals to take responsibility for risk taking in the complex world of modern medicine where lines between "treatment" and "experimentation" are blurred.

The malpractice suit involving Denton A. Cooley, a world-famous heart surgeon, clearly illustrates the limitations of the informed-consent doctrine. In this case, in 1969, Haskell Karp, a man from Chicago with a ten-year history of cardiac problems, was referred by his physicians to Dr. Cooley. After a week in the hospital, Mr. and Mrs. Karp met with Dr. Cooley, who recommended a heart transplant; Mr. Karp rejected the suggestion. A week later Dr. Cooley suggested a wedge procedure, an operation to remove destroyed heart muscles, and Mr. Karp signed a consent form specifically designed for this operation; it authorized cardiac surgery with the distinct possibility that a mechanical device might be used. The consent form read: "In the event cardiac function cannot be restored by excision of destroyed heart muscle and plastic reconstruction of the ventricle and death seems imminent, I authorize Dr. Cooley and his staff to remove my diseased heart and insert a mechanical cardiac substitute."[56]

By the time Mr. Karp was on the operating table, he was described by the physicians as "near death." The wedge resectioning was attempted, but Dr. Cooley inserted a heart pump in order, in his view, to prolong Mr. Karp's life. Mr. Karp thus became the first human to have an artificial heart implant. Dr. Cooley then sought a heart donor. Meanwhile, Mr. Karp's life was sustained by the artificial heart pump implanted in his chest. Within three days (64 hours) of implanting the artificial heart, Dr. Cooley found a donor heart and operated to replace the mechanical pump with a human heart. Mr. Karp died the next day.

While Mrs. Karp initially wrote warm letters of thanks to Dr. Cooley, she later decided to bring a lawsuit against him. She claimed that Dr. Cooley did not inform Mr. Karp that the device was experimental. The court looked at all the testimony, including the written consent form signed by Mr. Karp authorizing the artificial heart, and held that there was no basis for liability.[57]

Was the court correct in stating that there was no basis of liability? In one sense, the court's decision in *Karp* v. *Cooley* is not surprising if the informed-consent doctrine is seen only as a contract. According to the medical testimony, Mr. Karp was nearly dead before the operation, so it is reasonable to assume that he took the risks of the operation and the implantation of the mechanical heart (in light of the written consent) in order to save his life. If the purpose of liability rules is to guard against incompetence and to ensure that the individual patient assented to the inherent risks of the medical procedure, the court was undoubtedly correct in concluding there was no possible basis for liability. Dr. Cooley was probably the most competent heart surgeon in the United States, and Mr. Karp clearly intended to lead a more active life despite his many previous heart attacks and other cardiac problems.

But much larger issues are involved in this case than the court's analysis of liability rules would allow us to see. The court's analysis assumes that the transaction between Dr. Cooley and Mr. Karp involved only the two of them. This assumption allows the court to ignore the larger social context in which the wedge operation, the implantation of the artificial heart pump, and the transplant took place. Dr. Cooley was operating on the frontiers of knowledge. His techniques, using the latest in scientific research, should be seen in the larger context of heart research and cardiac surgery.[58]

Once we recognize that the procedure was experimental, we should realize that the biomedical research enterprise is necessarily involved in the case. We might assume that human participation in research is justified by patient consent, but such a perspective ignores the fundamental transformation that has occurred from the patient's perspective. Patients, even those with as serious a condition as Mr. Karp, enter the hospital hoping for a cure. Mr. Karp appeared to long for total restoration of his normal activities and seemed unprepared to accept a completely altered life-style. When the medical enterprise moves from its strictly healing function to experimentation, the patient needs some sign of this transformation, even though from the perspective of Dr. Cooley and his staff the difference between treatment and experimentation was essentially blurred.

Had the court recognized that the patient was to be offered an experimental treatment—a heart pump and transplant—it could have determined that Dr. Cooley ought not to have been the sole individual responsible for determining whether the device should be tried in a human for the first time. There should have been some social mechanism to assess the technical capacity of the device as well as its appropriate use. Some type of institutional review should have been required by the court. That is to say, before Karp could be asked to consent to the use of the mechanical pump, some group or groups within the hospital should have sanctioned its use in a human being.

Liability rules could be used to force hospitals to establish such institutional previews of new medical devices. The court could have suggested that the hospital, rather than Dr. Cooley, was potentially liable to Mr. Karp, if it did not have adequate means of reviewing research protocols before offering them to its patients. Such a rule is not too burdensome; all hospitals receiving federal funds already have such institutional review boards required by federal law.[59] Dr. Cooley's transplant program operated outside those constraints because his work was totally supported by private sources.[60] Given this anomaly, the court could have used liability rules as a means of encouraging the hospital, as an organization, to take responsibility for the various medical functions carried out under its auspices. The court's rule need not have suggested that the hospital adopt every aspect of the federal guidelines (for they are admittedly imperfect),[61] but it should have required some guidelines for human research. Such a requirement would have provided society with some reassurance that a social institution had considered the implications of the artificial heart implantation in all its moral, economic, and social dimensions.

Without institutional controls, Dr. Cooley (or any other surgeon, for that matter) is allowed to play the role of "lifesaver" without benefit of a specified social context. In his testimony in the case, Dr. Cooley explained that Mr. Karp's heart was so deteriorated that the wedge resection could not have been beneficial. Rather than stop at that point—a possibility if the larger context was made to influence his decision-making—Dr. Cooley proceeded with the operation because, he said, "We were under this obligation. I felt a moral obligation to try. We tried the wedge procedure and it failed. He ostensibly died on the operating table, so we proceeded with the alternative."[62]

Some might applaud the heroic and noble role that Dr. Cooley envisioned for himself when he implanted the heart pump in Mr. Karp. Similarly, Dr. William C. DeVries, who, along with his colleagues, designed the heart pump and connected it to its first human recipient, justified the entire project in essentially moral terms: "Heart disease continues to exact the greatest toll of human life, causing approximately one million deaths each year in the United States."[63] We must remember, however, that it is still not clear that the artificial heart program is a socially desirable path to pursue. After the first few replacements of a human heart with a mechanical device, we should remind ourselves that many treatments are technically feasible but not necessarily useful.[64]

Chapter 2

Hospitals, Mental Hospitals, and Other Caretaking Institutions

Just as hospitals and mental hospitals need to be analyzed as primary organizations within the institution of medicine, medicine itself needs to be viewed as just one component of the broad social construct of caretaking. By placing these organizations within the broad social goal of caring, law can make decisions that link medicine's role to the caretaking functions of other institutions in society, such as the family and the nursing home. The following three lines of reasoning will show why law should view medicine as but one of society's caretaking institutions.

First, law needs to distinguish between lawsuits against physicians and lawsuits against hospitals. In analyzing a case involving experimental research within a hospital, it will become clear that the current legal analysis of monitoring the doctor-patient relationship is inadequate for taking into account the hospital and its various purposes—treatment, training, and research—before resolving conflicts generated from within the organization.

Second, it is time to recognize that medicine shares a social-control function with law, as highlighted by a controversy that brought into question the ability of an involuntarily detained mental patient to give an informed consent to experimental psychosurgery. In recognizing the realistic function of social control, law should prevent such experimental procedures, not because individuals who are detained lack the capacity to consent but because medicine has gone beyond its appropriate function of social control when it attempts to use medical approaches in dealing with problems more appropriately reserved for prisons.

Third, we will address three troubling legal conflicts—withholding treatment, compelling treatment, and deinstitutionalization—which call for the recognition that other caretaking institutions are more appropriately suited to address these issues than is the law. These other caretaking institutions include prisons, nursing homes, and, most importantly, families.

Experimental Research in the Hospital

In the summer of 1963, two physicians associated with the renowned Sloan-Kettering Institute and Cornell University Medical College were pushing the frontiers of knowledge in cancer research. Their central hypothesis concerned the immunological systems of cancer patients. One feature common to all cancer cases was an apparent inability of the human body to reject cells foreign to that particular organ or part of the body. One of the physicians had previously published a report in a leading scientific publication indicating that patients with terminal cancer rejected transplanted live human cancer cells at a slower rate than healthy humans.[1] The two physician scientists were aware of a number of possible explanations for the difference. Their report pointed out that the debilitated state of the terminally ill cancer patients, as much as the presence of cancer itself, could lead to the weakened immunological response indicated by the slower rejection of the live cancer cells.

Drs. Chester M. Southam, a full-time member of the staff at the Institute and an associate professor at Cornell University Medical College, and Arthur Levin, his research fellow, sought to answer the question raised by their published report: Did the general debilitation associated with serious illness lead to a weakened immunological response in the human body?

They began by seeking patients who had serious illnesses other than cancer.[2] As practicing physicians, they knew that such potential subjects were located in many New York City hospitals. Their search led to the Jewish Chronic Disease Hospital. Through personal acquaintances of Dr. Levin, Dr. Southam was able to discuss with people affiliated with the hospital the need for immunological studies on chronically ill patients without cancer. The executive director of the hospital referred the research team to Edward Mandel, chief of medicine at the Jewish Chronic Disease Hospital.

Dr. Mandel discussed the pilot study with several members of the hospital staff but, in the end, chose a resident physician named Deogracias B. Custodio to assist the research team. (Before selecting Dr. Custodio, Dr. Mandel also discussed the proposed research project with Drs. Avir Kagan, who held a position as coordinator in the Department of Medicine, Perry M. Fersko, also a coordinator in the Department of Medicine, and David Leichter, coordinator of medicine in charge of cancer therapy and research.) Dr. Mandel agreed to allow the research team, with the assistance of Dr. Custodio, to conduct a pilot study that consisted of injecting live cancer cells into twenty-two patients at the Jewish Chronic Disease Hospital. During the discussions with the research team, the question of whether the researchers would obtain written permission from the patients was raised and dismissed. Southam described the injections as "routine" tests; he also pointed out that similar injections of cancer cells were done to test the immunological response of all postoperative cancer patients on the gynecological services of two hospitals with which he was affiliated without obtaining the patients' consent.[3]

News of the pilot study spread throughout the hospital. In late August, Solomon Siegel, the hospital's executive director; Dr. Samuel Rosenfeld[4]; and Mrs. Minnie Tulipan, director of welfare at the hospital, heard about the project. At least one newspaper reporter called the hospital with inquiries about the experiment. On August 27, Drs. Kagan, Fersko, and Leichter, submitted a joint resignation to Siegel citing their objections to the experiments. In early September, a special meeting of the Medical Grievance Committee of the hospital reviewed the circumstances surrounding Dr. Southam's research project. The committee approved the project, reasoning that under the hospital constitution Dr. Mandel, as director of medicine and of medical education, had the authority to conduct a pilot study without prior review by the hospital's Research Committee. Moreover, the committee accepted the resignations of Drs. Kagan, Fersko, and Leichter. At its meeting at the end of September, the board of directors of the hospital, with only one director dissenting, approved the report of the Medical Grievance Committee.

By winter, William Hyman, the dissenting director, had filed a lawsuit against the hospital asking for the medical records of the patients involved in the research project. Hyman's suit would ultimately reach the highest court in the state.[5] The majority of the judges on that court eventually agreed with Hyman and ordered the hospital to give him copies of the medical records (with patients' names deleted to protect their legal right to confidentiality). By this time, the hospital had changed its own rules to require the written informed consent of patients involved in experiments, but the court ruled that this new policy did not obviate the director's right and duty to determine the truth concerning past practices not in accordance with the newly announced policy.[6]

Three of the seven judges dissented, however, arguing that there were unique facts surrounding the case that should prevent the medical records from being turned over: the state administrative agency in charge of investigating the professional conduct of physicians was involved in the matter, and the district attorney was aware of the experiment. In other words, the dissenters argued that other legal agencies—the state disciplinary agency and the local district attorney—and another organization, the Jewish Chronic Disease Hospital itself, were better equipped to offer a social response that directly dealt with the problem that was before the court.

The dissenters' view has an initial attractiveness because their suggestions highlight the court's failure to offer any solution to the conflict between those who thought the experiment was a noble and harmless step toward finding a cure for cancer and those who felt the experiments were similar to the atrocities committed by the Nazis. If you do not have a definitive solution to a deep moral dilemma, the dissenters seemed to reason, why not simply abstain and allow other agencies to offer one?

Professional disciplinary proceedings condemned Dr. Southam for his "unprofessional conduct" as a physician, but apparently the biomedical research community did not see this as relevant to his appointment five years later to lead the American Association for Cancer Research. The lawsuit, though generated by the controversy within the hospital about the experiment, did not offer any statement about the experiment's legality or morality. As we shall see, the judicial pronouncements were unclear as to the legal parameters of the doctor-patient transactions because of the narrow perspective that the judges brought to the lawsuit.

If we look more closely at the effect of the lawsuit on the hospital as an organization, the initial attractiveness of the dissenting judges' view wanes. In 1963 most people, including members of the medical profession, envisioned the hospital as an organization with one primary purpose: the treatment of patients. Under this conception, the central figure was the physician. Although many hospitals participated in training programs for physicians beyond their medical school education, these trainee physicians were "doctors" as far as patients were concerned. At the time, biomedical research, including clinical research, was not considered a clearly defined and distinct function of a hospital, particularly one such as the Jewish Chronic Disease Hospital.[7]

This view of the hospital supports the image of the physician as healer that so dominated our perception of medicine twenty years ago. Under this view the hospital had no effect upon doctor-patient transactions except to support whatever the doctor, and perhaps the patient, determined was in the patient's best interests.

What appears most significant about this case was the demonstrable lack of procedures by which a member of the organization could complain about the ethical propriety of the experiment. Moreover, the confusion that is apparent in the records was caused by a failure on the part of the participants involved to recognize that the various functions the hospital performed had changed their idealized image of doctor-patient transactions.[8]

The courts were thus faced with an organization unaware of its own social importance, not only as a place of treatment but also as a site for biomedical research and the training of medical personnel. Consequently, no policy statements came from the board of directors on the issue of informed consent in patient experimentation. The view of the client as patient was so pervasive that the hospital's top administration did not realize that clients could also be research subjects or training material. These roles, of course, do not convey the same positive moral connotations as does the role of patient. While moral ambiguity is inherent in various types of biomedical research, it is nonetheless the backbone of modern medicine and should be recognized as such and handled within the organization of the hospital. An explicit recognition by the hospital that research is one of its functions can, in itself, provide a protection against the moral risks inherent in human research.

The lawsuit filed against the Jewish Chronic Disease Hospital was about the relationship of the hospital as an organization to its patients as clients. Even though many of the facts used to persuade the court concerned doctor-patient relationship standards, this particular lawsuit actually sought to hold up the hospital-patient relationship for social scrutiny. In effect the suit posed two questions: What does a hospital as an organization owe to its patients? What kind of controls should directors of hospitals impose upon medical professionals in order to ensure that the organization performs its social functions?[9]

The hospital, of course, was collegial in its mode of operation in that power and authority were presumed to be shared among professionals. Still, the medical professionals involved with the experiment did transform the patients into research subjects, while assuming that their relationship could be governed by the traditional ethics of medicine. The organizational structure in which this admittedly subtle transformation took place revealed an inadequate structure for accommodating the various interests of treatment and research. In particular, the constitution of the hospital allowed the director of medicine to initiate pilot studies involving patients without requiring him to consult with any other persons for sixty days, at which time he was then obliged to consult with the Research Committee. That prerogative was, in itself, defective because the so-called pilot study had no safeguard. It was therefore legitimate for the law to interfere in the corporate affairs of the hospital in order to protect the patients' rights. By so doing, the court recognized research as a legitimate function of hospitals but required hospitals to provide some measure of internal protection to ensure its proper social functioning.[10]

Patients want the benefits of the science of modern medicine to be used in their particular cases but fail to see the physician as related to the scientist.[11] Hospitalized patients see the role of the physician as that of healer. Physicians may want patients to become realistic and objective about the fact that there must be research to reap the benefits of medical science, but it is appropriate for law, rather than physicians, to determine whether a certain procedure is experimental or should be classified as a treatment.

This line of reasoning, which considers the context in which the doctor and patient encounter each other, helps to define the function of courts when examining doctor-patient transactions. Furthermore, this approach highlights the role of other legal agencies, such as state disciplinary bodies, as well as the importance of delineating the role of research in medicine.[12]

Since 1966, federal regulations have required that informed consent be obtained from subjects before research can be undertaken.[13] These regulations apply not only to biomedical research but also to social science research. This social response to situations such as those described in the Jewish Chronic Disease Hospital case might be thought to provide a cure to the problems presented; however, studies indicate that the effectiveness of the written requirements is questionable.[14] One reason these consent reforms fail is that they do not consider the dominance of the hospital as an organization in doctor-patient transactions. Legal requirements for consent are also doomed to failure because sharing uncertainties with patients, subjects, or clients is generally contrary to the professional ethos of physicians and modern professionals.[15] The hospital, with all of its attendant anxieties about illness and abandonment, is the reality in which the sharing of information between patients and physicians occurs—or, more precisely, fails to occur.[16] Rather than look for solutions to the problems raised by the Jewish Chronic Disease Hospital case by further refining the legal requirements of consent, necessary as those requirements are because of our respect for self-determination, we might look at the way in which law perceives the hospital as an organization and medicine as a social institution.

Medicine and Social Control

In the early 1970s, another group of physician scientists were attempting to advance the frontiers of knowledge about the human body. Ernst A. Rodin, a neurosurgeon, and his associate, J. S. Gottlieb, a psychiatrist of the Lafayette Clinic in Detroit, Michigan, were investigating the nature of human aggression and violence. Their hypothesis was that uncontrollable aggression might be the result of brain malfunctioning, which could be corrected or altered by certain surgical techniques developed by modern biomedical research.[17] Drs. Rodin and Gottlieb sought to carry out an experiment to test their hypothesis, but the proposal alone led them into litigation. This litigation, known as "The Psychosurgery Case,"[18] has been scrutinized by national commissions and the mass media over the years.

The original purpose of the research project was to compare "medical versus surgical treatment of patients who have been committed to the state hospital system because of severe uncontrollable aggressive outbursts."[19] In other words, certain individuals were supposed to receive drug treatment for their socially unacceptable aggression while others were to undergo a form of brain surgery.[20] The researchers' proposed study was based on recent literature indicating that some spontaneously aggressive individuals suffered from brain abnormalities. Removing areas of the brain scientifically determined to be the cause of the behavior had led in some instances to fewer and less violent outbursts in patients with epilepsy. From this published work, the researchers reasoned that some of the patients in mental hospitals might also have brain abnormalities which would respond to similar treatments. Thus a control group of patients was to receive an experimental drug that would reduce the level of the hormone testosterone, on the theory that this hormone was "in all probability" responsible for aggressive behavior. An equal number were to undergo brain surgery.

The proposed study had two notable features: the researchers were relying on the published work of noted authorities,[21] and they were trying to apply this research to a new area of great social concern. In addition, they assumed that drug treatment was preferred to surgical treatment because of its relatively low cost and effective delivery.

Included within the proposal itself were several devices designed to guard against the risks inherent in the experiment. First, the proposed implantation of deep electrodes to study the brain patterns and the actual surgical removal of any portions of the brain would be done at hospitals affiliated with the department of neurosurgery at the local university medical school. This stipulation implied that those most experienced with the new techniques would be involved. Second, the researchers established a committee of medical specialists who would examine all the medical charts of potential patients from the state hospitals in order to guard against surgical operations being performed on those without extensive abnormalities. This committee would conduct a scientific and medical review of the researchers' own medical judgments concerning which patients' abnormalities were appropriate for surgical removal (since many abnormalities are not). Third, physicians serving on the medical review committee formed another committee, consisting of a clergyman, a law professor, and a community representative, to guard against infringements of patients' rights and to review the consent forms that were signed by the patients and their families. Finally, the researchers established an additional control in the form of a list of criteria to ensure that the patients selected were not only the most likely to benefit from the experiment but were also the ones who might be viewed as the most appropriate risk-takers. (Patients with certain psychiatric disorders were excluded, for instance.) These criteria included the requirements that the patients had to be male, over twenty-five years of age, with IQs above 80, residing in a state hospital for at least five years, and regarded as untreatable by conventional means. The controls made sure not only that psychosurgery was the only known hope for these patients but also that, if "cured," they would have a chance of functioning in society. To buttress their position the researchers mentioned that the state legislature had funded the project, indicating that the proposed study was considered to be of sufficient social importance to deserve state support.

The proposal was stopped when a lawyer associated with the local legal services agency found out about the project, informed the press, and brought a lawsuit halting the experiment. By the time the lawsuit was filed, only one person had signed a consent form; after the ensuing publicity, even this potential patient and his family withdrew consent. The state funds allocated for the project were also withdrawn. The lawsuit was continued, nonetheless, on the grounds that the issue was deemed important enough to merit a declaratory judgment. Although the two researchers dropped their plans, they continued to express belief in the basic appropriateness of the study.

The court condemned the experiment on several grounds. With references to the Nuremberg trials, the court ruled that an involuntarily detained person could never consent to the type of surgery proposed because it was essentially experimental. The court relied upon the familiar argument that involuntarily detained mental patients would be subject to subtle coercive pressures from the fact of their incarceration. Physicians have greater status and power than their patients, and this inequality, along with the fact of incarceration, led the court to prohibit the surgery until such time as it could be viewed as treatment rather than experimentation.[22] Furthermore, the court had already ruled that the patient who signed the consent form was illegally detained in the state mental hospital and had to be released. The court reasoned that he was being held in the hospital under a statute that was itself illegal. The man, referred to as John Doe to protect his right to anonymity, had been incarcerated in a mental hospital for seventeen years for the alleged rape and murder of a student nurse. He had been committed without criminal proceedings under a statute labeled the Criminal Sexual Psychopathic Law, which the court held unconstitutional.

In its long and confusing opinion, the court implied that it was morally inappropriate for medical professionals to try to isolate the biological factors that determine human behavior. Yet the court did not consider whether it would be appropriate to try to isolate the social and environmental factors involved in human behavior, particularly aggressive behavior. What appears to have motivated the court was the notion that medicine is concerned solely with treatment, and that the law's duty is to ensure that protected classes, such as prisoners and mental patients, receive the benefits of treatment while being protected from experimentation.

I recognize that biomedical research is a critical part of modern medicine, but I would argue that the proposed psychosurgical experiment should still have been canceled, and on grounds other than lack of informed consent. Viewing the detainee more like a prisoner, the court could have held that experimental psychosurgery was "cruel and unusual punishment."[23]

It is important to recognize both the similarities and the differences between the medical experiments of Dr. Southam and Dr. Rodin. Both research groups were tackling problems that raise fundamental questions in modern biology: Dr. Southam was trying to unlock the mystery of the human body's immunological response; Dr. Rodin was trying to understand which neurological and possibly biochemical reactions in the human brain cause certain types of behavior. Both groups had turned to hospitals to find the appropriate research subjects.

One important difference, however, is the hospital each used. From a biomedical viewpoint, a mental hospital is not a "real" hospital. The dissociation of psychiatry from the organizations in which it is practiced is based partly on the position that, unlike hospitals where treatment takes place, psychiatry seldom cures its patients.[24] The view of psychiatry and mental hospitals as separate from medicine is also based on a scientific and moral critique: psychiatric treatment is often not subject to laboratory confirmation of results, as is most of modern medicine. The x-ray film reveals whether a bone has healed, for instance, but how does one determine if a deep depression has ended when a patient is discharged from a mental hospital? Under this exclusionary view, it is thought best to link psychiatry to some other institution in society, such as religion. The moral criticisms of psychiatry are concerned that the most difficult cases require compulsion in the form of involuntary hospitalization. Psychiatry, therefore, does not meet the ideal of the voluntary doctor-patient transaction.[25]

The most striking dissimilarity between Dr. Rodin's attempted project and Dr. Southam's is that Dr. Rodin's research required a great deal more social scrutiny before it could be conducted, while appearing on the surface to be within the mainstream of the traditions of scientific medicine. Partially because of society's change in attitudes toward human research, Dr. Rodin's project was encumbered with many more procedures designed to protect human subjects. Yet despite these procedures, Dr. Rodin's research project led to litigation.

Medicine has long been a part of social control, and this role has been dramatically created through development and use of the mental hospital. We can, in a sense, view mental hospitals as organizational structures through which modern medicine makes its contribution to restoring mental health.

What has not been said in everything written about the alleged problem of psychosurgery is that law and medicine are both instruments of social control. Medicine's mechanisms of control are built within hospitals and thus provide the governing structures for modern doctor-patient transactions. Law's social-control functions in relation to medicine are attempts to regulate the parameters of the institution of the hospital and define the minimum social obligations of physicians as professionals. The positive social function of medicine is that of restoring health to members of the community. It is in this role and in caring for the sick that medicine shares its caretaking functions with other institutions in society.

The Caretaking Function of Medicine

In the practical world of modern medicine, physicians are enjoined by cultural precepts, including law, to take care of patients. Caretaking is defined as protecting the best interests of patients and providing them with the basic requirements of life: food, water, and shelter. This caretaking function is crucial to understanding many legal and medical encounters. At an institutional level, medicine's caretaking function is so widespread that we consider any social ills that require caretaking to be within its jurisdiction. Institutions for the mentally retarded are a prime example of organizations infused with this medical ethos, although it is not clear whether any medical cures in the traditional sense can be attained. A number of other institutions also provide caretaking in a generic sense and thus share with medicine some caretaking functions in society. These include nursing homes and families, which—at least with respect to children—are expected to provide the care necessary not only to sustain life but also to protect the health of their members.

The caretaking function of medicine and its relationship to other caretaking institutions in our society are best illustrated by examining three legal developments. The first revolves around the issue of withholding medical treatment. The second concerns the authorization of treatment against the expressed wishes of the patient. The third deals with attempts to deinstitutionalize patients currently in mental hospitals and facilities for the mentally retarded.

Withholding Treatment

From a mentally retarded man. Joseph Saikewicz, sixty-seven years old and severely retarded, was discovered to have an incurable form of leukemia. His case presented two additional problems that made him a difficult patient: his mental retardation was so severe that he was unable to speak, communicating with others only by gestures and grunts, and his IQ was estimated to be 10; according to the court's opinion, he had a mental age of two years and eight months.[26] In other words, by the time his case came to court, Joseph Saikewicz was a "silent patient."[27] Furthermore, those members of his immediate family who could be contacted expressed no interest in attending the hearing that would decide the course of his treatment. Thus, no one provided the physicians with traditional family support in dealing with a life-threatening condition. Saikewicz had effectively become a ward of the state; the state institution had become his parent.

The lawsuit technically began when Saikewicz's caretaker, the superintendent of the institution where he lived, asked the court to appoint someone other than himself to decide whether potentially life-prolonging treatment should be administered.[28] After a hearing in which the judge listened to the testimony of the attending physicians and the attorney for the state institution, the judge agreed with the recommendation of the court-appointed guardian that Saikewicz should not receive the normal treatment, chemotherapy, for his form of leukemia. While several legal doctrines were discussed by the judges who heard the case, the court essentially decided that, in Saikewicz's case, the possible good results of efforts to prolong his life were not worth the adverse and unpredictable effects of chemotherapy.

The court arrived at this remarkable decision with repeated disa-
vowals that it was based on the perceived quality or lack of quality
of Saikewicz's life. The physicians, for instance, informed the court
that Saikewicz would, in all probability, have to be restrained in
order to receive the intravenous treatments that could affect his
"success" potential. The court admitted that some of the medical
testimony about the ability of older patients to withstand the side
effects of chemotherapy was, at best, questionable[29] and that Saikewicz did not understand the reasons for the treatments or his pain. The
court also admitted that there was a "low chance at producing
remission."[30] Nonetheless, the judges, lawyers, and physicians involved seemed convinced that it was in Saikewicz's "best interests"
to die rather than endure the pain of chemotherapy treatments.

The question of withholding treatment would be difficult to answer in any sixty-seven-year-old patient with an incurable form of
cancer, but, until recently, very few persons would have thought
legal intervention could help the situation. Given the complicating
factors in Saikewicz's case, one suspects that legal intervention was
sought not in search of greater wisdom but as a way of sharing
professional and moral responsibility about law and medicine's caretaking functions.

The definition of a facility for the mentally retarded and the duties
it is expected to fulfill are at the core of this case. The court in
Saikewicz may have assumed that the institution for the mentally
retarded shared the same broadly defined goals as the hospital for
cancer treatment, since both institutions are frequently called hospitals. The function of mental retardation facilities—actually called
hospitals in some states—is as unclear and varied as are the reasons
for placing individuals in them. In the traditional sense a mentally
retarded person is not someone with a disease that can at present be
"cured." At best, conditions of mental retardation can be ameli-
orated by positive social and medical intervention, but at worst,
living in a state institution for the mentally retarded can cause a
deterioration of the patient's condition.[31] Such institutions become
places that care for those for whom families and the other institutions in society are either unwilling or unable to provide.

In addition, Saikewicz's fate was shaped by the prospect that, were
he to enter a hospital for cancer treatment, his grunting, gestures,
and possible physical restraint would prove disturbing to the professionals who have an image of the "good patient." Although all
doctors would agree abstractly with the proposition that the hospital
ought to care for its patients, Saikewicz appeared to require too much
care. In a sense, he was a patient that medicine as an institution
wanted to reject as unsuitable, since other social institutions, particu-

larly the family, had already relinquished responsibility. Medicine's caretaking function seems to take for granted a readily available supporting mechanism outside of itself, which cares for the patient's health and thus shares its goal. Such a support mechanism appeared lacking in Saikewicz's case, and this lack may explain why he was rejected for treatment.

Despite the support of other caretaking institutions, such as families, there may be deep conflicts between them and modern medicine because of their differing views of what health means. When lawyers and judges are asked to arbitrate these battles concerning the health of a person whose life is at risk, there is the additional complication of the legal concept of health, which is also slowly changing in face of the new realities of medicine. Nowhere is this type of conflict more dramatically illustrated than in cases that involve withholding treatment for children and newborns.

From a child with Hodgkin's disease. When Joseph Hofbauer's parents refused to follow the advice of his attending physician to consult a specialist in oncology or hematology for treatment of his Hodgkin's disease, a form of cancer that afflicts the lymph glands, they were sued by the local government for neglect. The parents had taken Joseph to Jamaica, where his disease was treated by nutritional therapy, including injections of laetrile. Unlike classically neglectful parents, the Hofbauers were acting upon their belief that there were better alternatives to restoring Joseph to health than the conventional treatments of radiation and chemotherapy.[32] Eventually Joseph and his parents returned to New York and found a physician licensed in the state who shared their belief in metabolic treatment for cancer. This physician also indicated in the court proceedings that he would recommend conventional radiation and chemotherapy if the metabolic treatments were not proving successful.[33]

Despite metabolic treatment, Joseph Hofbauer died a year after the litigation began.[34] His death seems particularly painful to those committed to conventional medicine's healing image, because there is some hope of remission through radiation and chemotherapy for those who suffer from Hodgkin's disease.[35] On the other hand, the side effects of the proposed conventional therapy rejected by the parents—including a possible later cancer—are so varied and unpredictable that it can never be recommended without caution. The prospect of death in Joseph's case makes one want to compel the parents to risk the side effects of radiation and chemotherapy. But the court, when faced with caring parents who rejected conventional treatment in favor of alternative methods, sided with the parents. In its reasoning, the court paid deference to conventional medicine by suggesting that since the parents had taken Joseph to a physician licensed in the state, they could not be found neglectful.[36] In its opinion, the court seemed to be suggesting that any conflict within medicine about the appropriate treatment for cancer was not within law's domain to resolve. Thus the court cannot be criticized for failing to impose the risks of chemotherapy upon Joseph against his parents' wishes, unless one believes that judges have the power to make a quality-of-life assessment in weighing one treatment against another.

To resolve the court's dilemma would have first required the recognition of the importance of science to modern medicine. The court did so to a limited degree by taking expert testimony from a biologist, in addition to physicians, about the effectiveness of metabolic treatment for cancer. But the court did not comment on the larger issue of the costs of delay from conventional medicine's perspective.

This decision probably left the treating physician and most conscientious physicians with the feeling that law has no understanding of the importance of medicine as an institution when faced with a conflict of values with the family. In the classic forensic approach to issues of medicine, the judge was entitled to accept the evidence; however, he did not realize that the standards of evidence in law and science are considerably different. Had the court recognized that the causes of cancer are unknown and that therefore a range of experimental treatment is viewed by practicing physicians as acceptable, it could have provided some guidance, but not direction, to Joseph's caretakers. At the time of the trial, metabolic treatment was clearly experimental: that is, not acceptable as conventional treatment by the overwhelming majority of professionals. Before Joseph's parents, as his caretakers, could authorize the nonconventional treatment, the court should have instructed the scientific and institutional committees within the hospital to conduct a review. These committees should neither have the power to prevent the proposed treatment nor be expected to be morally wiser than the parents. Instead, they should provide the parents with information, acting as a source with no direct stake in the outcome.

In point of fact, the Hofbauer parents were in conflict not simply with the conventional view of cancer treatment but also with the conventional or objective view of health.[37] This particular case for the withholding of conventional treatment, when presented to law for resolution, revealed a deep conflict in values about the meaning of health. Health is variously defined by caretaking institutions, families, and institutionalized medicine, and these differences are exacerbated by recent biomedical advances, which have forced all members of society to reevaluate their own concepts of health.[38]

From a baby with spina bifida. In performing the appropriate social function of law, courts can be helpful in resisting attempts to impose one view of health on everyone, as occurred in one portion of the Baby Jane Doe litigation.[39] Here the New York court resisted an attempt by a concerned outsider (a proponent of the Right to Life Movement) who was neither a parent nor a state welfare official to force the parents to submit Baby Jane Doe to surgical treatment for spina bifida. After consultation with medical specialists, nurses, and their own religious counselors, the parents elected instead to pursue a course of treatment that meant probable death within two years. By dismissing the suit, the court simply gave the parents as the baby's caretakers the right to make that decision.

This allocation of responsibility is particularly appropriate in making health care decisions for newborns, since recent medical advances have made so many more choices possible. To force a particular treatment risks imposing the medical profession's view of health upon all individuals in the society. The predominant view within the profession might be to attempt surgery "in appropriate cases," but this does not mean that an individual physician would hold this view when faced with a particular patient. It is likely that professional norms would encourage the surgeon to go forward. By listening to parental doubts about the value of surgery and choosing not to operate, the physician would be finding good reasons for not following professional expectations. To force a particular treatment upon the parents of a seriously deformed newborn, in effect, gives a supreme place to medicine's caretaking functions, a place above all others in society.[40]

Compelling Treatment

Both nursing homes and prisons are institutions that must care for their clients in a generic sense, but until recently the issue of whether law should be used to compel treatment within these institutions was not a matter of public discussion.

At one level, the issue of compelling treatment of patients who also happen to be prisoners appears somewhat straightforward. The jailer can be seen as the caretaker of the prisoner, whose liberty to seek medical treatment, unlike other citizens, is restrained.[41] But when the prisoner refuses proffered treatment, one might fall into the trap of suggesting that the loss of liberty involved in incarceration allows the medical profession to ignore the prisoner and speak to his caretaker, the jailer. Such an analysis fails, in part, because medicine is recognized to be of such overriding importance in society that a person has some claims on medicine, as a patient, that may override his status as a prisoner. Usually these claims are phrased in terms of the prisoner patient's consent, which is generally thought to be an important issue of medical ethics.

For a prisoner with kidney disease. A case where a prison warden asked a court to compel treatment of a prisoner who had refused kidney dialysis illustrates the role conflicts that medicine must face.[42] It is surprising that the same court which allowed the withholding of treatment in Joseph Saikewicz's case found legal doctrines to justify the compulsion of dialysis treatment in this case (even though, strictly speaking, dialysis is not a cure for the underlying kidney disease). It is also surprising that the medical profession participated in this compelled treatment. At the level of what courts now call medical ethics, one might wonder why the physicians were willing to go along with the legal fiction that there is consent when the prisoner involved was competent, but could have been using his lack of consent to dialysis as a means of obtaining goals relating to his imprisonment.[43] In the Saikewicz case, for instance, the physicians expressed concern about the possible necessity of physically restraining the patient in order to administer chemotherapy, whereas in the case of the prisoner the physician seemed anxious to carry out his moral duty and use physical restraint if necessary to "treat" his patient with dialysis.[44]

Given the scarcity of dialysis machines, one wonders why the physician was not more hesitant in offering this treatment to a reluctant patient. There are three reasons for the willingness of physicians to participate in the compulsion of hemodialysis. First, physicians have not traditionally been asked to make the decisions themselves about who should receive treatment and who should not (and, in the case of hemodialysis, who should die). We have taken political steps to ensure that the scarcity of machines and the ensuing allocative decisions are invisible to the physician through federal insurance for dialysis.[45] As far as the attending physician was concerned, there were no other patients who needed that particular dialysis machine.

Second, since medicine serves a caretaking function, it is perhaps easier than we like to acknowledge to proceed without consent. This is particularly true since the warden was himself a caretaker accustomed to proceeding without this patient's consent in various penal situations. Coercion in health care matters is generally directed toward the restoration to health of all members of the community. We are not neutral toward illness; we make it plain to the patient that the socially desirable thing to do is to "get well." In other words, coercion is more endemic to medicine than we care to acknowledge, and we find only certain forms of coercion in medicine objectionable.

Third, the caretaking institution seeking the physician's help was itself a legal institution designed for social control. Since medicine is a part of the social-control network, it could relatively easily become allied with prisons, since such an alliance would only strengthen medicine's role.

For those who will not eat. The willingness of medicine to participate in compelled treatments is demonstrated by the response to a prisoner who simply refused to eat as an act of political protest. Providing food is the simplest of any caretaker's duties, so it is a good way of looking at the caretaking function generally. When such a situation arose in Northern Ireland, the English courts did not intervene to authorize force-feeding. In the United States, however, law and medicine would probably authorize forced intravenous feeding if the patient were a prisoner,[46] since the state's caretaking role in prisons is sufficiently broad to allow for it.

Although little attention is given to the issue of force-feeding prisoners in the United States today, the force-feeding of nursing home patients has become a matter of public debate and lawsuits. If nursing homes are defined as places of caring for the critically ill rather than as caretaking institutions for the dying, law should not condone the refusal to force-feed nursing home patients. Nor should law establish the "right" of a nursing home patient to stop forced feeding as a way of resolving this public debate. Rather, we should recognize that we have equated "treatment" with "caring" and have fallen into this intellectual trap because we have too easily accepted the role of medicine as preserving life rather than as caring for patients.[47] We have assumed that nursing homes are part of the institution of medicine without reflecting on the ancillary but distinct role that nursing homes perform.

We need some method of distinguishing the role of treatment for the critically ill from the role of caring. Although caring for patients is always required, treatment may be appropriately withdrawn when the proper group—family, doctors, nurses, friends—makes the difficult decision that treatment is no longer in the patient's best interests. Law helps society make this distinction by refusing in many instances to decide nursing home cases brought before it.[48] By refusing to decide, legal decision-makers, primarily judges, must make clear that nursing homes should have their own policies to resolve such questions as the removal of feeding tubes. The suggestion that hospitals classify patients in terms of the level of treatment needed ought to be applied to nursing homes, although the residents would still be classified only in terms of the type of medical treatment they required.[49]

Deinstitutionalization

The term "deinstitutionalization" has been generally applied to efforts to have patients in large state mental hospitals—and, more recently, residents in large state facilities for mentally retarded persons—moved to smaller community-based facilities or returned to their homes.[50] In the litigation that has developed around the issue, confusion has grown about the functions and goals of deinstitutionalization. Many confuse the policy of trying to develop smaller-scale facilities with the treatment itself. (It is as though we expect a person who has spent five years in a state mental hospital to be "cured" by being released.) Although it is commonly understood that anyone released from a large state institution will require considerable care, it is surprising how few communities, particularly urban communities, have been able to provide the type of care required. New York City is often cited as a prime example of the failure to provide for the newly released, but it is no different from many other cities in this country and abroad.[51]

Up to now the litigation in this area has not clarified the issues of caretaking that are involved in deinstitutionalization. With regard to mentally ill patients, law is still in a quandary trying to decide if patients who have been involuntarily committed for treatment have a legal right to define the form of the treatment.[52] This litigation suggests the whole question of whether one can separate the caretaking function from the treatment function. In the case of mentally retarded patients, attempted deinstitutionalization has tragically reached the limits of human capacity to care. As these cases work their way through the courts, we hear official caretakers, such as parents, asking for relief from the burdens of severely retarded family members. More recently, we have witnessed suits asking state administrators of these facilities to provide the legislatively mandated "treatment and care" for residents, even those without any prospect of release.[53]

In a recent suit, the litigants, former patients in large state mental institutions, asked the court to compel the state to provide them with "a home."[54] This suit was filed against the background of a need to build new organizations—often called halfway houses—to provide care. We have not asked ourselves why society has not provided enough halfway houses or social support outside the large state mental hospitals that everyone claims to abhor. Unfortunately, we have been unable to recognize the need for institutionalized care in society; we have tended to romanticize these halfway houses as "homes" and have failed to provide the institutionalized protections for them through law. Law cannot force an individual to care for another person in a private sense.[55] It can only recognize the limitations of institutions and provide the context for caretaking. Such a context implies restrictions on those who run caretaking institutions such as hospitals and on physicians.

It is all too easy to blame medicine for the tragedy that deinstitutionalization represents. We fail to see the limits of medicine because we believe in its unlimited capacity to cure. We too easily assume that "care" and "cure" are axiomatic without realizing that our capacity as a society to care has been impaired. This is most dramatically seen in the case of mentally retarded children, where society has been unable to provide the necessary support for the official caretakers, their parents, to encourage them not to abdicate full caretaking responsibilities in favor of state institutions. If society's tolerance for the mentally ill or the mentally retarded could be magically increased, the need for large-scale institutions would be diminished. Instead, we are more likely to ask medicine, the youngest science, to assume caretaking responsibilities for our most difficult cases.

Chapter 3

Specialization and the Physician's Social Obligations

Specialization is one of the defining characteristics of modern medicine. As a result, when individuals enter the health care delivery system, they are often referred to specialists.[1] But specialization is not simply a method of organizing modern professionals. It is also a way to think about knowledge and thus a way to resolve social problems.

In analyzing the social obligations of physicians from an institutional perspective, I shall discuss the battered child syndrome, administrative regulations of the neonatal nursery, and a psychotherapist's liability for failure to warn third parties of the potential danger of his or her patient. The effect of specialization in medicine is now so pervasive that law, in many instances, has accepted the expertise of medicine without fully exploring its implications for social problems.

In analyzing law's attempts to cope with the medical and social risks of highly specialized treatment, I shall discuss the legal regulation of electroconvulsive therapy. Although existing attempts at direct regulation of specialized treatments are faulty, law has an important social role to perform by providing patients with a means to question the organization and financing of modern health care.

The Nature of the Physician's Social Obligations

To battered children. The scene is a hospital emergency room. One of the patient's legs has a spiral fracture; there are bruises over her entire back as well as superficial abrasions over other parts of her body. In performing his diagnosis, the examining physician wants to know something about the origin of the injuries. The patient in this case is eleven months old, so the inquiry is directed to her mother. The mother is silent or says, "I don't know."

What should the physician do in face of the evidence before him? The child has certain serious injuries that he can categorize according to his medical training; however, he does not know the causes of those injuries, which might affect the manner of his diagnosis and treatment.[2] Besides the medical facts, he has one crucial social fact: the patient's mother, her primary caretaker, claims not to know how her daughter was injured. Professional guidelines exist to help the physician. Moreover, the organization within which he is performing his duties, the hospital, ought to provide some guidelines, even if those guidelines simply adopt the standards of the medical profession. Examination of these and other sources for the physician's normative behavior might provide some insights, but they do not address the question of the physician's social obligation in a direct manner. In fact, there are limitations on the ability of the hospital and the medical profession to define the social obligations of the physician.

Law stands in awe of medicine at the same time as it seeks to impose its structure upon it. Law has a picture of medicine's social obligations, and in that context it imposes sanctions upon medical professionals and hospitals for failing to live up to that imagined standard. Medicine, perhaps from an awareness of its own impact as a social institution, quite often develops medical categories that embody social phenomena. The categories used to define mental illnesses are examples of this, just as the battered child syndrome is another medically developed category that contains both medical and social features.

The situation of this eleven-month-old patient comes from a California case dealing with the battered child syndrome.[3] This term, coined by Dr. C. Henry Kempe, refers to a collection of symptoms and injuries in a young patient that were intentionally inflected by someone else. The term combines two notions: first is the medical concept of "syndrome"—a collection of symptoms, much like the idea of toxic shock syndrome. Then there is the highly emotive suggestion that the child has been assaulted and beaten. The medical and social course of action for the attending physician has been charted in a landmark article by the physician who coined the term.[4] Having established that such symptoms as fractured legs and bruises are part of the battered child syndrome, the physician is supposed to make an assumption about the social reality of the situation and then proceed.[5]

To recommend a social course of action would require the physician to develop a model of adult-child relationships. Dr. Kempe suggested that successful "treatment" involved notifying the police or a child protective agency. This appears to be a reasonable course of action, since the intentional injury may be an indication of criminal behavior and a child protective agency would need to become involved with the case. Since Dr. Kempe assumed a battering parent frequently continues to assault the child, notifying the police also may protect the child from further injuries. Implicit throughout his analysis is the idea that the battering adult may be in need of help, may in fact be mentally ill and in need of medical attention.[6] Thus the conscientious physician would seek not only to heal the wounds of the child but also to remedy the social fabric of the family.

But if the physician fails to recognize the collection of symptoms as the battered child syndrome or recognizes the syndrome but does not wish to become involved with the police and child protective agencies, certain social sanctions besides those of professional criticism or censure can be brought to bear. All states have provided legislation that requires physicians to report cases of injuries involving a possible violation of the law, especially cases of child abuse, to the police and other authorities.[7] Failure to report would mean the physician has committed a crime. Using this legislation as a background, the California courts maintained that the physician who failed to report could be held liable for professional negligence.[8] Subsequent injuries to the child by the battering adult are viewed as the legal responsibility of the physician, based upon the assumption that additional injuries could have been prevented through appropriate action. As a result, law, in addition to imposing criminal penalties, might require the physician to pay monetary damages for failing to report child abuse.

On the one hand, a court's willingness to base a civil liability suit on the failure to recognize the battered child syndrome means law has adopted the implicit social reasoning involved in Dr. Kempe's article. In effect, the courts are saying that any physician not versed in the battered child syndrome is operating below acceptable social standards regardless of the quality of the treatment he or she may have provided for the perceived injuries. The physician is potentially responsible for injuries that were not detected and the additional injuries the child patient might receive later. The imposition of liability against the physician is thus a recognition of the importance of protecting the life and health of children in society.

On the other hand, the ultimate effectiveness of the legal tools that the potentially liable doctor is supposed to invoke leaves much to be desired. The prevailing child protection statutes in the United States are based upon the assumption that the battering parent can be treated for the supposed mental affliction that leads to the battering and can thus be healed by modern medical intervention. Modern child welfare statutes also assume that there has been no irreparable damage to the child, apparently because the physical injuries have received proper medical attention. If either or both assumptions are, as I suspect, unwarranted, does liability for the physician who fails to invoke the legal system make sense?

The evidence we have—although much needed data, such as the amount of sexual abuse of children, are simply unavailable—indicates that the battered child is permanently damaged, both psychologically and emotionally.[9] But the legal implications of these studies have been the subject of great controversy. Present child welfare statutes have focused on the physical health of the child and the mental health of the parent, since the battered child syndrome identifies both as possible patients. If, however, the child protection statutes focused solely on the physical and mental health of the child, law would require the removal of the child from the parent.[10] Moreover, if the child protection statute were clearly child centered, the case for imposing an affirmative duty upon the physician to report battered-child cases to the authorities would be stronger.

At present, law reflects a certain ambivalence about and perhaps false hope in the power of modern medicine. Law is reluctant to impose what some judges would see as a penalty against the abusing parent by permanently removing the child. Social service provisions for the abusing parent are based on the hope that there is the capacity to "cure." In this sense, the image law has of medicine is highly wishful and, by most accounts, unrealistic. Without denying that some parents might be "cured," it must be accepted that these battering parents view the love of their children in a socially confusing way. Most parents take their assaulted child to medical authorities without even suspecting that such serious injuries are likely to lead to criminal prosecution.[11]

At present, this legislative attempt to define the social obligations of physicians fails because the legislatures have not articulated the background social conditions for imposing a positive duty upon physicians to involve police and other state officials. We should bear in mind that in this society (but apparently not in civil-law countries like France or West Germany) the law does not usually impose civil or criminal liability on the failure of individuals to act, because in law there is no general social duty to help or care for others. (Under our laws, a person who fails to rescue a drowning baby is not criminally liable, with one exception: if the person is the child's parent, he or she is criminally responsible for the child's death because of the social and legal duty of the parent to protect the health of the child.)[12] Physicians, despite their special position in society, are normally not sanctioned for their failure to accept a patient or prevent harm to a person; thus, the imposition by law of a social sanction for their failure to protect a battered child from further harm is questionable, unless there is a clear social duty. Without certain kinds of child protection legislation, the social duty of a physician remains unclear since the legislature has not clearly defined the obligations of members of society at large, including parents, to refrain from injuring the child or suffer legal consequences.

One might think that any legislative attempt to define the social duty of the physician in a situation of child battering might fail because legislatures do not have sufficient expertise to provide guidance in an area that requires both technical and moral judgments. Given the complexities of medicine and the rapidity of developments, one might argue that administrative agencies are better equipped to delineate the social obligations of physicians. But even administrative agencies can define their authority only in relation to social assumptions underlying legislative action.

To newborns. Thirty years ago there were no neonatal techniques to use in a case such as Baby Jane Doe, born with severe deficiencies in her spinal cord that affected her entire nervous system,[13] as described in chapter 2. The surgery option offered to her parents did not promise to remove or improve her handicapping conditions but gave only the possibility of prolonging her life. Under such circumstances, the role of law should be to encourage decisions that preserve our now evolving notions of life and to threaten or impose sanctions on those who make medical decisions contrary to a clear social consensus that a particular life is worth preserving. After an individual from the Right to Life Movement failed in the state courts to obtain an order forcing the hospital to perform the surgery,[14] a federal administrative agency, the Department of Health and Human Services, brought suit against the hospital. The basic contention of the federal government was that the patient was a "handicapped individual" who might have been denied medical treatment in violation of federal law. The government claimed it needed to examine the hospital records to determine whether or not the hospital had engaged in unlawful discrimination.

While no one would deny that Baby Jane was a "handicapped individual," the court nonetheless held that the statute covering unlawful discrimination was not intended to apply to medical decisions involving newborns, where the parents had refused to consent to medical intervention.[15] Underneath all its reasoning about the myriad statutes and administrative regulations involved in the case, the court held, in effect, that the administrative agency had exceeded its authority. The court was correct in its assessment. The background social consensus was insufficient to force the hospital either to proceed with the operation without parental consent or to seek an order in state court to perform the operation.

The background social consensus can be illuminated by discussing whether the parents or the physicians would be criminally liable for failure to treat Baby Jane Doe. As just noted, the usual rule in Anglo-American law is that one is not responsible civilly or criminally for failing to act unless there is a special relationship that imposes a clear social duty to do so. In Baby Jane Doe's case there existed the special relationship of parent and child. But the notion of social duty was established at a time when medicine did not have its present capacity to sustain newborns and when the injunction to attempt cure in every case was an operative guideline for physicians. Baby Jane Doe's medical condition in light of present knowledge probably destroys the once clear social duty to have the surgery performed.[16] There obviously are members of society who strongly believe that surgery ought to be performed in cases such as Baby Jane Doe's, as well as those who support the parents' decision not to have it. Both sides could argue their position reasonably, and that is enough to destroy the notion of a clear social duty.[17] Even if there is confusion surrounding a physician's social duty, however, there is no guarantee that criminal liability might never be imposed by a jury.

If parents are to remain the primary decision-makers, hospitals ought to encourage them to consider their attachment to the newborn and the hope that it represents, as well as the realistic outcome of any proposed treatment. Most modern neonatal nurseries have achieved this type of structure by providing a setting in which parents have almost unlimited access to their newborn child and its medical caretakers, thereby providing some assurance to society that they have considered all the factors in arriving at their decision regarding treatment. The properly organized neonatal nursery can counteract the notion that there is only one objective and scientific solution to be reached.[18] Within the proper hospital setting, physicians can fulfill their social obligations of presenting parents with the options for treatment. The newborn at risk should never be shut away from its parents, because it is not the function of the physician to treat the newborn as a dying patient. Nor is it the physician's social obligation to treat in every case. Rather, it is the physician's duty to join with parents and nurses in making difficult decisions under circumstances of uncertainty.

To violent psychiatric patients. Moving from the technologically sophisticated and morally complex setting of the neonatal nursery to the armchair of the psychotherapist, one might think it would be easier for law to define a physician's social obligations. But in the case of a young graduate student who expressed the wish to kill a fellow student who had refused his romantic advances, one might easily assume that the physician is placed in a situation similar to that of the physician examining the battered child. Under such an assumption, the physician would be expected to determine the likelihood of such threat's being carried out, while proceeding to aid the patient and to protect the supposed victim by notifying the authorities, if warranted. As there is no landmark piece of writing for psychotherapists that identifies a collection of symptoms and gives recommendations on the treatment of the violent patient comparable to Dr. Kempe's battered-child article, one might assume that the physician has the obligation to use his or her judgment in keeping with the professional and legal rules on the confidentiality of medical records, particularly psychotherapeutic records.

If the threat is carried out, however, a court could define the social obligations of the psychotherapist without consideration of the background social conditions of law and medicine. Such was the case in *Tarasoff* v. *Regents of the University of California*, [19] where the California Supreme Court held that a psychotherapist had a duty to warn a victim of his patient's possible violence. The court relied in part on the Principles of Medical Ethics of the American Medical Association to suggest that the psychotherapist's obligation of confidentiality should yield to public safety when disclosures in general are allowed under the AMA principles. The court did this, based on its hope that danger to the public could thus be averted. [20]

In the *Tarasoff* case, the therapist involved was not technically a member of the medical profession but rather a psychologist working under the supervision of a psychiatrist at the university's health center. In fact, many persons who practice psychotherapy are not medically trained; psychologists, social workers, ministers, and others often practice some form of psychotherapy. The court does not explain why the general standards of ethics for physicians should apply to a psychologist. I suspect that the court was probably so taken with the model of medicine as scientific healing that it would place any professional engaged in alleviating any form of human suffering under the standards of the American Medical Association. By so doing, the court assumed that a psychologist's assessment of a patient's potential to carry out a threat of violence is analogous to a physician's diagnosis of a standard medical disease. Thus if a physician has a clear duty to see that harm to the community is averted, it would appear logical to insist that a psychotherapist, who might be thought of as someone who specializes in the potential for violence, must also see that harm to a possible victim is averted. [21]

A person who voluntarily seeks out a psychotherapist is seeking help with some emotional, social, psychological, or spiritual problem. Until these types of concerns lead to social dysfunctioning, the client will not be hospitalized. Up to that point the person represents no greater threat to the social fabric than any other person, although there may be difficulties for those with whom the person lives and works. In this context hospitalization is significant because it is a background condition a court can use in defining the social obligations of the psychotherapist. Hospitalization indicates that the community has been unable to heal or restore the person to health, for whatever reasons. Hospitalization also means that the psychotherapist-patient relationship has changed its context from an office practice to a hospital-centered one. In this sense the psychotherapist-patient relationship becomes more like a doctor-patient relationship, since the hospital organization provides a social context in which the modern biomedical ethos of medicine plays a significant role in the treatment.

In many cases that psychotherapists treat, hospitalization is significant because law has provided for the possibility of compulsory hospitalization. When considering the issue of a patient's potential for violence, nearly all states in the United States and most Western countries have laws requiring the committal, even if it be involuntary, of patients who pose a danger to themselves or others. But almost no state or Western country allows an adult to be involuntarily committed solely for the purpose of treatment.[22] Law has already decided when the individual patient-psychotherapist relationship ought to be brought into the larger social context by allowing the therapist, if he or she also happens to be a licensed physician, the official authority to invoke the institution of the hospital without the patient's consent.

Under such an analysis, the result of the Tarasoff case—holding the therapist liable for failing to warn a possible victim of his patient's potential danger—is ironic at best. The psychotherapist had attempted to have the graduate student involuntarily committed but had been overruled by his superiors. Because he was not a physician, he did not have the authority to commit his patient without the consent of his superiors. Only a physician or qualified psychologist is supposed to be able to judge when a patient is dangerous enough to justify hospitalization.[23] Furthermore, given the confidentiality of the psychotherapist-client relationship, it was merely fortuitous that the victim's family gained any knowledge that the murderer had been undergoing treatment with the therapist.

So far, the court has not been willing to hold a therapist responsible for the self-inflicted death of a patient.[24] At the very least, the court should have noted that the effect of holding responsible the clinical psychologist, who had no ultimate authority in the clinic or within the law to bring about the commitment, is to decrease the role of psychologists in the delivery of mental health services. This reduction has been brought about without considering that the role of medicine is to help the community preserve the health of its members. When courts are asked to define the social obligations of a highly specialized professional, such as a psychotherapist, they have to take into account these background social conditions in their attempts to reconcile the traditional notions of the doctor-patient transaction with the wider social responsibility of medicine.

Referral to the Specialist

The patient, a professional woman in her early fifties, has come to the physician complaining of fatigue, loss of appetite, weight loss, and an inability to sleep at night. A careful examination and questioning does not reveal a physiological cause for the patient's problem. After prescribing a conventional tranquilizer, the physician arranges to see her again after a short period of time. As the patient's condition worsens and her ability to perform normal social duties continues to be impaired, the physician diagnoses her condition as deep depression and refers her to a specialist, a psychiatrist, who may try a number of treatments, such as drugs or certain forms of psychotherapy, which could involve the patient's husband.

When the patient's depression persists, the psychiatrist recommends a period of hospitalization in a private psychiatric hospital, concluding that the deep depression she has experienced for nearly a year has led to her total emotional and physical exhaustion; she needs rest to deal with the causes of the depression. In the private psychiatric hospital she is prescribed rest along with other forms of therapy. After nearly two months in the hospital, her psychiatrist and others involved in her treatment conclude that her condition has not improved; a more radical treatment must be considered.[25]

If the form of depression that the patient has is endogenous or chemical, she might be considered a candidate for electroconvulsive therapy, in which electrical current is passed through the brain, inducing convulsions.[26] Despite the risks involved, such a treatment would be considered for two reasons: the social realities represented by a particular case and the relative effectiveness of the treatment. Given the patient's age, unless she can be restored to social functioning within a few months of her hospitalization, there is a great risk of her becoming a permanent hospital patient.[27] And if left untreated, her condition could lead to suicide.

A conscientious psychiatrist would consider electroconvulsive treatment (ECT), despite popular images of it, because of its medical effectiveness. At present, ECT is reserved for patients with chemical depression who do not respond favorably to drugs. When ECT is used as a last resort, from 70 to 90 percent of depressed patients respond favorably, meaning that their severe depression is "cured" or treatment is continued on an outpatient basis.

It is impossible to determine which patients will respond favorably, however, because the biological basis for explaining the effectiveness of electroconvulsive treatments is poorly understood.[28] In addition, there are some well-documented side effects of ECT, not all of which can be guarded against.[29] Moreover, the electrical stimulation of the brain leads to cognitive disturbances for which there is no means of prevention. In the short term, nearly all patients have temporary amnesia and confusion. A small number of patients experience a longer memory loss, disturbing many facets of their lives.[30]

Such adverse reactions, coupled with the inexplicable nature of the success of ECT, have led many to suggest that law should regulate its use. Since no evidence is available about the long-term effects of electrical stimulations to the brain, the call for regulation is based primarily upon the "mind altering" and possibly dangerous effects of ECT. To introduce legal regulations would be somewhat ironic since all normal precautions required by law are generally taken by conscientious electroconvulsive therapists. In my hypothetical case, the patient and her husband would be asked to assent to the treatments. Though they both hesitate in the face of the known risks, which have been explained to them in detail, in the end they decide that the potential social gains of restoring a professional woman and spouse to the community outweigh the risks.[31] This situation illustrates several issues that arise from specialized medicine.

Most intrusive treatments, particularly those likely to cause legal concern, are performed by specialists rather than primary-care physicians. As a result, the patient has gone through a series of referrals in order to establish the correct diagnosis and proposed treatment. The significance of this for ECT patients is twofold. First, the patient is no longer with his or her primary-care physician or health care professional, traditionally regarded as a healer, but rather with a highly trained specialist who is accustomed to dealing with "difficult" cases and may be more of a risk-taker than the average person. Where the patient may still be looking for a cure, the specialist may have a different definition of successful treatment.

Second, because of the risks involved, the specialized treatment takes place within the hospital. Within that setting there is the social possibility of long-term commitment to a mental hospital, something viewed as socially undesirable by laymen and professionals alike.

From both a medical and nonmedical point of view, we prefer to see persons with diagnosed mental illnesses outside the hospital. Contrast this with the heart surgery patient. Although the goal of restoring social functioning of the patient is the same, there is a less dramatic social backdrop of potential changes in life-style of the patient and the effects of those changes on the family. With both the heart patient and the ECT patient, we would prefer to see the patients alive and using medicine to prevent the perceived risks to life. The major difference may be that with the heart patient we assume that the patient and the surgeon have the same goal, but with the ECT patient, given the nature of the illness, we are less certain that the patient shares the physician's and society's preference for life.

Specialized medicine is partially a function of the growth in biomedical knowledge. This has a particular significance for ECT. In general, physicians have an incentive to narrow their area of practice and so improve their competence in areas where biomedical knowledge is expanding. In ECT, only those physicians whose professional sphere is closely aligned with the treatment are likely to administer it. These physicians, who are both researchers and practitioners, attempt to heal those whom other professionals cannot, giving evidence to the claim that specialized medicine is both pragmatic and altruistic.

Law helps to increase the tendency toward specialized medicine by penalizing those who fall below a certain standard and by increasing the regulation in the practice of medicine. Opinions such as in *Tarasoff,* where the physician who fails to predict the violent behavior of a patient can be held legally responsible, should encourage physicians to refer those patients with a potential for violence to specialists. For those procedures perceived as risky, law has tried to impose a regulatory scheme. In ECT cases, several states have passed statutes requiring greater supervision in the taking of "consent."[32] These statutes reflect society's view that other values are at stake when medicine seeks to alter the brain, and perhaps the etiology of the illness itself is outside the province of medicine, even though there are few other means of coping with deep depression.

If risks were the only consideration, the attempt at regulation of ECT makes no more sense than an attempt to regulate consent in open heart surgery, but these efforts help to focus our attention upon an underlying problem: How do we judge whether highly specialized medicine is more "efficient" than less-specialized medicine?

The difficulty in dealing with medical specialists is that patients are understandably always concerned with individual aspects of health. From a social perspective, the general health of the community must also be considered in any judgment of highly specialized medicine.

The general view of the community includes its feelings about proper care for the "sick" with highly technical and sophisticated forms of medicine. Given the growth of knowledge in medicine, we are not likely to revert to a practice of generalists as opposed to specialists. Therefore, we must allow for the development of alternatives to specialized medicine in seeking a definition for the health of the community. In this regard law has a useful role to play, not by direct regulation of the practice of certain specialized techniques such as ECT but by an overall regulation of the referral system that tends to monopolize the notion of health. Law can, in effect, place legal restrictions on physician referrals. Three cases aptly illustrate the social role law can play in highly specialized medicine.

In the first case, a person brought an antitrust action against a group health plan that paid for psychotherapy performed by psychiatrists (who are licensed physicians), but not for the same treatment performed by psychologists (who are not). The group plan would reimburse for treatment by a psychologist only if that treatment was supervised by a psychiatrist and the bills were submitted by the physician. In upholding the right of a patient to bring a suit under the antitrust laws,[33] the court was in effect allowing the patient to have some role in defining the delivery of health care services. While the court upheld this right by regulating the financial structure used to pay for medical care in America—third-party reimbursement— the court was implicitly defining medicine as an institution. This point can be elucidated by considering the implication of a contrary ruling. This would mean that the physicians and the third-party insurance company could decide the way in which certain health care needs would be met. Thus without knowing it, the court was saying that the structure of health care delivery is not solely the function of institutionalized medicine.

In the second case, the federal government brought a successful action against the AMA for its code of medical ethics, which limited the contractual arrangements between physicians and nonphysicians and placed restrictions on physicians in advertising the price of their services.[34] The effect of this opinion is to restrict the role of the profession in structuring the delivery of health care. While it may be important for physicians not to consider the dollar cost of health care from the perspective of traditional medical ethics, costs may be an important factor for individual patients in evaluating their own health care.

This type of litigation has been followed by a third type of case, lawsuits filed by a state against the American Medical Association, the American Hospital Association, and other professional organizations to eliminate their restraints on the practice of chiropractors.[35]

This final case has two implications: first, that the legislature, not the institution of medicine, has the authority to determine the types of medicine that can be practiced in the state, based on the principles that the function of medicine is to protect the health of the community and that the definition of health is not one profession's exclusive view; second, that by restraining hospitals and other professional organizations from discriminating against chiropractors, the court is giving these professionals access to the predominant organizations and referral systems of modern health care delivery.

This third case might raise objections on the ground that legislators ought to protect the public from chiropractors, whom most physicians view suspiciously, because of an apparent lack of scientific support for their practice. But conflicting notions of health are, in fact, part of the present social context of doctor-patient transactions. Law's function is not to preserve prevailing notions of health but to allow for the evolution of the community's particular notion. Within that context, modern medicine can continue to make its contribution by providing health care services to the community without using law to destroy alternative views of health and, by extension, alternative ways of organizing health care professionals.

Conclusion

As a result of the growth of specialization in medical practice, law needs to redefine the social obligations it places on physicians. The institutional approach suggests that the social obligations of physicians ought to be seen in the larger context of how law has generally defined the obligations of persons in our society. With this approach the legislative requirement that physicians report evidence of child abuse raises the larger question of whether law has clearly defined the obligation of parents to care for and preserve the health and lives of their children. Once it is apparent that law's response to the parent who abuses a child is ambiguous, wholesale adoption of the social assumptions behind the medical category called the battered child syndrome is unwarranted.

Administrative agencies have been no better than legislatures in attempting to define the obligations of physicians in relation to children. These regulations adopt the prevailing perspective of attempting to supervise the doctor-patient relationship by trying to override the traditional requirement of parental consent to treatment for severely impaired newborns. These regulations were correctly struck down by the courts as long as there remains the possibility that the parents' and the physicians' social obligations could theoretically be tested through criminal prosecution and neonatal nurseries are structured so that a parent has continued opportunity to care for his or her impaired child.

Courts themselves, however, have failed to analyze law's obligation to prevent violence when imposing liability upon a psychotherapist who did not warn a third-party victim of the danger from his patient. The court too easily assumed that its image of the obligations of physicians should be imposed on psychotherapists, whose numbers include many helping professionals with different training and ethos from physicians. Furthermore, the court might have assumed that the psychotherapist was a specialist in preventing violence without considering the operative effects of such an assumption on the delivery of care to socially dysfunctional persons and the use or misuse of mental hospitalization.

Courts, however, are the best agency to help law come to grips with the implications of specialization. Courts should resist legislative attempts to overregulate specialized care such as electroconvulsive treatments, despite the risks inherent in those treatments. Furthermore, courts should resist the attempts of modern medicine to use its authority and power to structure the delivery and financing of health care in a manner that places alternative concepts of health and of the organization of medical professionals at an economic disadvantage. Through these efforts, courts could then encourage members of society to focus on the fundamental question of whether highly specialized medicine is better for society than less specialized medicine.

Chapter 4

Caring for
the Critically Ill

With the growing success of modern medicine in treating disease and the development of more sophisticated methods of emergency care, heretofore private issues have increasingly become matters of public discussion. One result of this heightened public interest in the fate of the critically and terminally ill is that courts have begun to play a major role in monitoring the decision-making of the family members, friends, professionals, and organizations involved in these cases.

There is an increased push for a well-established legal "right to die," based on the premise that justice would be served if the authority of the patient to decline treatment was clearly established. In response to pressures such as these, courts have used the idea of the patient's right to decline treatment to resolve the ethical issues surrounding the critically ill. But so far they have failed to develop either a moral consensus or even an agreement on legal procedure. Furthermore, recent court decisions purporting to bring order and certainty to the confusion of the present situation have only rendered the lack of a moral consensus even more apparent.

The current judicial analysis does not take into account the larger institutional context of medical decisions, including the inherent uncertainty of those decisions that may result in death. The culmination of these judicial developments is the suggestion that legislatures ought to establish procedures for implementing the right of individuals to decline treatment under all circumstances, including their possible future inability to communicate. This idea, popularly known as a "living will," is an attempt by adults to declare in advance and in written form what medical treatment should be proscribed in the event of certain conditions.

In my view, legal recognition of the "right" of an individual to be the sole moral decision-maker in medical matters does not provide caring or justice for the critically ill in the context of hospitals and nursing homes. Three kinds of cases will illustrate how recent court opinions dealing with terminally ill patients conceptually lead to the individual patient, even when comatose, as the sole decision-maker about the course of treatment or nontreatment.

The first case involves the question of whether family members' definition of death should prevail over an institutional definition put forth by medicine and law. By imposing a brain-death definition in that case, the court opinion upholds the premise that there is an objective and medically correct decision about death that law can impose when faced with a critical illness.

The pair of cases considered next suggest that evidence in a document similar to a living will should be legally and morally determinative in resolving conflicts about treatment of critically ill patients. By authorizing the withdrawal of treatment on the basis of whether the critically ill and "silent" patient has left some evidence that courts can use—specific objective evidence about the course of medical treatment—this opinion ignores the role of *caring* as opposed to *treatment* of the critically ill. The mode of discourse about caring, which involves nonverbal communication, must be discovered by law. For when a person indicates a preference for no *medical treatment,* law should not assume that this person, or even one who has expressed no preferences, does not desire *care* for his or her illness.

The last case, referred to briefly in chapter 2, involves the question of whether a feeding tube can be removed from a nursing home patient at the request of a relative. In deciding the relative's request, the court developed a set of procedures aimed at trying to understand the nursing home resident's intentions regarding feeding tubes or other medical assistance. In developing its elaborate procedures for dealing only with nursing home as opposed to hospital patients, the court missed an opportunity for discussion of the role of the judiciary in the context of nursing homes as caretaking institutions whose functions are distinct from hospitals.

The institutional focus on these cases will reveal that death, as part of the much larger concept of health, must be viewed primarily as a social rather than biological state that law simply confirms. By viewing death as social as well as relational, we will begin to see that caring for critically ill patients involves personal involvement—emotional, spiritual, and psychological—rather than the objective distance implied in our present use of the term "health care." Law, were it to adopt this institutional focus, would see that legalizing living wills as the solution to the dilemma of caring for the critically ill is counter to the long-term goal of bringing about some form of social harmony.

Definitions of Death

The first case involves Alex Haymer, who was seven months old when his parents took him to the Foster G. McGaw Hospital. Critically ill, he was placed in the pediatric intensive care unit and attached to a mechanical ventilation system. Subsequently, a pediatric neurosurgeon examined Alex and determined that he was "brain dead." The neurosurgeon's diagnosis was confirmed by two other physicians. The hospital then sought to remove the mechanical ventilation system, but Alex's parents objected. The hospital turned to the courts for a resolution of the dilemma rather than pursue other possible means of resolving the conflict.[1]

In accordance with prevailing medical standards, the court held that Alex died when his brain functioning stopped, not when his heart stopped a month later. The court reviewed the current medical and legal literature but failed to acknowledge fully the parents' and the court-appointed guardian's objection to turning off the ventilation system. The court assumed that the parents were relying upon the more traditional definition of death—the stopping of Alex's heartbeat.[2]

In its apparently cool and dispassionate application of legal precedents, the court failed to note the underlying irony of its decision; the case seems to imply that the prevailing medical definition of death—an objectively determined fact—supersedes any personal or subjective definition of death. Put more graphically, the case implies that the parents' view of the breathing baby as alive, albeit with mechanical assistance, is totally irrelevant if that view conflicts with the prevailing medical definition of death. A further implication of the case is that law will adopt without discussion prevailing medical standards about what is essentially a theological question. Such a legal posture cannot be deemed just, nor does it promote any notion of healing.[3]

The essential question remains of whether or not this was a conflict that the court, as opposed to some other body, should have resolved. One possibility, not considered by the court, was that it might have declined to decide when "death" occurred. While under some circumstances it would have been appropriate for the court to decide when Alex died, this was not the case here, since the suit asked solely for a declaration of rights, without a discussion of the nature of the underlying conflict. Granted, the idea of legal uncertainty is anathema to physicians and laymen who equate certainty in law with justice. But let us pause for a moment and analyze the nature of the alleged uncertainty that would have been caused by the court's refusal to decide when Alex died.

If there had been a suspicion of child battering, the physicians in charge of the case should have investigated the child's injuries according to existing medical and legal standards. This obligation to investigate applies whether or not Alex is dead by any standard. There is no evidence that the investigation was hampered by an inability to interview the parents about the cause of Alex's injuries—a part of the medical diagnosis in any case—or to take x-ray photographs of the child. If evidence exists to justify criminal charges of assault, for instance, there is nothing wrong with going ahead with the investigation, bringing charges, and later changing the charge to homicide if Alex dies. The hypothetical criminal investigation and prosecution is not hampered by Alex's status as legally dead or alive.

If, in the course of a criminal prosecution, the parents wanted to raise as a defense the question of the time or cause of Alex's death, the courts would then be in the proper position to adjudicate the question of whether brain death can be used in a legal setting (in this case, a criminal prosecution). But the more serious and obvious objection to my proposed approach is that the parents might sue the hospital or the physicians if the ventilation system were turned off without their consent. The fear of such a lawsuit is far greater than any likelihood of its success, especially if everyone else involved with Alex's case had agreed that Alex was dead. Whether or not there is evidence of criminal misfeasance toward Alex, the threat of a lawsuit encourages the physicians and the hospital administration to become engaged in a series of conversations with the parents to convince them of the correctness of the decision to remove the ventilation system. These conversations force the medical profession to articulate the underlying moral basis of its brain-death standard.[4]

If the parents tried to claim that Alex's death was caused by removing the ventilation system, the defense in a malpractice action would be that Alex was already dead. Such a defense would be asking the court to declare that the brain-death definition ought to be adopted in that particular state. The parents' contra argument would have to be based on some medical testimony. Provided there has been no negligence in handling the case, it is difficult to see how the parents could marshal the medical evidence to support their claim. There is always the theoretical possibility, of course, that a jury might react emotionally and award monetary damages regardless of the evidence, but such irrationality is uncommon and would only be a sign that the community at large had not yet accepted the prevailing medical standards. But the question of the legal definition of death is a matter for resolution by the court, not a jury. As a question of law, the entire issue of the appropriate legal standard of death could be decided by a judge before a jury even heard the evidence. If decided in accordance with the medical establishment's view, the case would be dismissed.[5]

The immediate legal risks, in fact, are quite minimal in Alex's case. The difficulty is long-term and system-wide. Lawyers and judges have accepted without question the idea that physicians and hospitals are entitled to total legal certainty in facing the moral problems occasioned by critically ill and terminally ill patients. This quest for certainty has not helped us resolve moral problems; it has only added to the confusion. Furthermore, this more activist posture of judges has led to a misconception of the function of law as a social institution because there has been no articulation of the role of courts and, by extension, the role of other legal agencies such as legislatures in relation to the institution of modern medicine. Alex's case is a good example of how law, unwittingly and without explicit discussion, can adopt an imperious view of modern medicine which may help to achieve some underlying moral certainty on the part of judges and lawyers but which generally adds to the level of confusion about what ought to be done.

The Living Will and Discontinuing Treatment

So far the prevailing solution to the moral problems encountered is to offer all decision-making authority to the individual patient, on the premise that the patient must consent to treatment and therefore has the right to decline treatment. But this simple principle becomes enormously complicated in practice, because the critically ill patient is often not capable of making treatment decisions. In an attempt to resolve this difficulty, legal commentators and judges have promulgated the concept that those involved in the health care decision should try to determine what the prospective intentions of the person were *before* he or she became critically ill. This concept underlies the growing popularity of the living will. In describing the background judicial developments for the idea of living wills, I shall comment on the way in which these developments reflect the prevailing confusion about the interaction of law and medicine.

Brother Fox

The highest court of New York was the first to state that decisions about discontinuing treatment would depend primarily on the patient's prior attitude. In order to develop this doctrine supporting the practice of making living wills, the court, in a single 1981 opinion, considered two cases together.[6]

In the first of these cases, the court considered whether an eighty-three-year-old priest could be disconnected from a respirator, once it had been determined that he had lapsed into a persistent vegetative state following cardiac arrest during an operation to correct a hernia. When the priest, Brother Fox, could speak, he told members of his order that his life should not be prolonged if he were ever in such a state. After learning that there was no reasonable chance of recovery for Brother Fox and after retaining two neurosurgeons who confirmed the diagnosis, the director of his order, Father Philip Eichner, requested that the hospital remove the respirator supporting Brother Fox's breathing. The matter became the subject of litigation when the hospital refused to remove the respirator without a court order.

By the time the case reached the appellate courts, there were two kinds of evidence. First, the medical experts called by the local prosecutor indicated that there might be some improvement in Brother Fox's condition. The medical condition of "persistent vegetative state" was a particular kind of coma and had already become the subject of litigation in the Karen Ann Quinlan case. All the medical experts agreed, however, that there was no reasonable likelihood that Brother Fox would ever emerge from his vegetative state and resume cognitive functioning. Second, testimony from members of Brother Fox's religious order indicated that under the circumstances he would want the respirator removed. He had expressed this view during a discussion his religious community had held on the moral implications of the Karen Ann Quinlan case. These discussions took place within the religious community, since it was part of the order's mission to teach and promulgate Catholic moral principles. Brother Fox apparently expressed agreement with papal teachings that consider the use of a respirator "extraordinary" means of sustaining life. Several months before he went into the hospital, Brother Fox had indicated that he would not want his life sustained by what he called "extraordinary business" if his condition were, in the court's words, "hopeless."

The court, paying very little attention to the medical testimony, used the lay testimony to establish several legal rules for dealing with health care decisions concerning terminally ill patients. The court held that where "clear and convincing evidence" of the patient's wish to discontinue a life-supporting system was available, as in the court's view there was in Brother Fox's case, a guardian of the adult patient had the authority to order the respirator removed. The court went on to hold that the guardian did not need prior approval from a court (as indicated in the Massachusetts cases, which will be discussed later). The court also stated that the authority to discontinue treatment was based on common law rather than on the constitutional principles cited by both the Massachusetts and New Jersey high courts. The important implication of the Brother Fox ruling was that a common law–based decision can be modified by the legislature, whereas constitutionally based rights cannot be diminished by legislative actions in the American legal system.

John Storar

The court used the principles established in Brother Fox's case to decide a second case, one that involved a conflict between the parent of a fifty-two-year-old profoundly retarded man with terminal cancer of the bladder, John Storar, and the state administrators of the institution where he lived. The question concerned whether or not the patient should receive blood transfusions. The mother, who was also the patient's legal guardian, had refused to consent to the blood transfusions on the grounds that they would only prolong her son's discomfort.[7] Rather than accede to her request as legal guardian, the hospital administrator applied to a court for an order to continue the blood transfusions, not to save his life but simply to postpone his ultimate death.

There were three kinds of testimony before the court, coming from a variety of sources. The medical testimony confirmed that Storar had terminal cancer, which, by the time of the hearing, had spread to his lungs and possibly other organs. His life expectancy was estimated at from three to six months, and he required two units of blood every eight to fifteen days to replace blood he was losing. Without the blood transfusions, he did not have sufficient oxygen in his blood and would become strained and lethargic, perhaps even bleeding to death. After the transfusions, he was more energetic for a time and able to resume his usual activities. Some of the medical experts testified that it was more appropriate at this stage of the illness to limit the treatment to only the administration of painkillers and to discontinue the transfusions, since they only prolonged the suffering.

There was further evidence pertaining to Storar's social and mental state. He had been in the residential facility since he was five years old. Some of the medical experts testified that he had the mentality of an infant of approximately eighteen months. There were also indications that he disliked the blood transfusions, apparently did not comprehend their purpose, and was also distressed by blood clots in his urine, which usually increased after the transfusions. Storar was given a sedative before the transfusions and was regularly given narcotics to help alleviate the pain that the physicians believed he was experiencing.

Third, there was the evidence submitted by his guardian, his mother. At the time, she was a seventy-seven-year-old widow who lived near the residential facility and visited her son almost daily. Storar was her only child. She stated that her goal was simply to make him comfortable, and from this perspective the transfusions were not justified. She also admitted that no one had explained to her what would happen to her son if the transfusions were discontinued. In addition to her confusion about the medical implications of her decision, she stated she could not determine whether he wanted to live, although she thought he wanted to avoid the transfusions.

The highest court found little difficulty in reaching the conclusion that the blood transfusions should be continued, basing its decision on principles outlined in the Brother Fox case, which emphasized the need for a clear expression of desire on the part of the patient prior to terminal illness. Since Storar was incompetent and unable to express any such desires, there could be no clear way to approve of discontinuing the blood transfusions based on his wishes. In looking for other principles, the court found that guardians should not be allowed to discontinue lifesaving treatment. In the court's view, the blood transfusions were lifesaving since they changed almost certain death within a few weeks to a three- to six-month prognosis. The court expressed sympathy for what it called the mother's despair but failed to discuss the relevance of her somewhat confusing testimony. So, while the court held that a court order was not needed in situations where there was a clear expression of the patient's will, it assumed the implicit authority to order the blood transfusions in John Storar's case.

Looking solely at the prognoses in Brother Fox's and Storar's cases, we see that the court was motivated by some overriding idea of the legal process. Brother Fox was a critically ill patient, but there was no clear prognosis of death as long as his breathing was assisted. The court noted that his condition was precisely the same as Karen Ann Quinlan's—a persistent vegetative state—but failed to note that Karen Ann was weaned from the respirator and continued to breathe, if not, from some perspectives, to live. Had Brother Fox not already died by the time of the court decision, removal of the respirator would have meant almost certain death. John Storar, on the other hand, was a terminally ill patient. He had undergone several months of treatments and there was, by the court's own admission, some support within the medical community for the mother's position. But the principle that the court was seeking to uphold is that of rational and unequivocal decision-making in the face of impending death.

This principle can be illustrated in two ways. On the positive side, the standard established in the Brother Fox case encourages individuals to formally declare their wishes before they are faced with a critical illness. Since most individuals do not belong to Catholic religious orders or other organizations that formally discuss these issues, the best way for them to make their intentions known is through a written document, a living will. It is clear from the court's decision that it wants a solemn and formal declaration of intentions.

On the negative side, Mrs. Storar's testimony was not given much credence because of her lack of understanding of the medical diagnosis. Her testimony and her actions—giving and withholding consent—demonstrate the ambivalence one might expect in parental attitudes toward terminal illness in a child. Her honesty in face of the unknown—she modestly admitted an inability to determine whether her son wanted to live (but testified to a perceived revulsion when the blood transfusion equipment was brought into his room and a marked increase in the amount of pain he seemed to be generally experiencing)—has no place in a legal system designed to pin moral responsibility for death within the medical context on one individual. The court is so intent on upholding the principle of prior individual decision-making that it implies in its opinion that no parent would have the authority to stop blood transfusions in the case of a child with terminal cancer. The strength of this implication is somewhat modified by the unspoken fear that Mrs. Storar may have had conflicting feelings about her son because of his severe retardation. There may thus be an unspoken desire on the part of the court to protect the mentally retarded from being not only placed in institutions but passively killed through neglect once they become critically ill.

This kind of attitude provokes public demand for the recognition of the "right to die." The court opinion seems to imply that medical procedures must be used in the face of terminal illness in order to maintain law's, and presumably society's, strong preference for life over death.

The court's handling of Brother Fox's case, of course, has led to a growing public interest in writing living wills. There are two problems generated by the case which need to be addressed. First, how did the court arrive at this particular posture? And second, can the living will be effective within the context of institutionalized modern medicine?

To understand how the New York court arrived at a result where the terminally ill patient—John Storar—could be forced to undergo ameliorative though noncurative treatment and the critically ill patient—Brother Fox—could be allowed to die, we must realize that the court has not thought systematically about its own role in the world of modern medicine. It has used its traditional role in resolving conflicts without considering whether institutional medicine requires some procedural innovations in law. As noted earlier, courts ought to be sensitive to the timing of their declarations on admittedly vague medical/legal concepts, such as when death occurs.

The majority of the court in *Storar* failed to note that the person bringing the suit, the acting director of the facility in which the patient lived, was not the proper person to bring a lawsuit compelling treatment against the wishes of the patient's duly appointed guardian. As one dissenting justice pointed out, the lawsuit should have been dismissed, without any discussion of the underlying substantive medical and ethical issues, on the premise that the residential facility, when viewed as a health care provider, lacked a substantial interest in the outcome of the litigation.[8]

Although individuals within the institution might care deeply about John Storar or believe strongly that they should resist attempts by those not involved in work with such persons to denigrate the quality of life of the mentally retarded, the court would not be entitled to take such a position. First of all, individuals associated with the institution who have strong moral feelings about Storar's treatment do have an opportunity to bring those feelings to bear on the situation. Individuals who have mentally retarded persons in their daily care exercise some influence by virtue of their greater knowledge of the individual and their role as the interpreter of the individual's experiences. When a visitor comes to the institution, the caretakers usually interpret what the resident has been doing, feeling, and experiencing, even when the visitor is the biological parent. In Storar's case, it is apparent from the record that when he became ill, the persons on the staff were able to convince Mrs. Storar to change her mind about diagnostic tests and blood transfusions on at least two occasions. Their ability to influence her was based both on their clinical expertise and their position as Storar's caretakers. Allowing the institution to bring this lawsuit gave the individuals within the institution another opportunity to impose their view of health on Storar and his legal guardian.

Second, had the court dealt with Storar's case by dismissing the lawsuit, it would have had a more consistent posture vis-à-vis its assertion in Brother Fox's case that, generally, courts need not become involved in health care decisions for the critically ill even when the decision may lead to the patient's death. But dismissal in the Storar case would have demonstrated an underlying fallacy in the reasoning of the court in Brother Fox's case. In dismissing the Storar case, the court would have had to explain that there are alternative means of legal intervention and that prior judicial authorization should be viewed as extraordinary rather than expected in any morally difficult situation. If, for example, members of the staff believed that discontinuing the blood transfusions offended some basic moral precepts, they could have asked the local prosecutor to investigate. That such an option seems not only distasteful but unlikely indicates that individual views on matters of major significance such as health are not generally given credence except when they are seen as having an effect on society generally. While individuals within the institution may be motivated by strongly held beliefs, I suspect that a lawsuit, once it is in the hands of the legal establishment, would at best be only an anticipatory defensive action on the part of the institution. The important procedural innovation would be a clear statement that only certain persons would have standing to bring a lawsuit to compel treatment over the objection of the patient or his duly authorized legal representative.[9]

Before the New York decisions, two other state appellate courts, New Jersey and Massachusetts, had written opinions dealing with health care decision-making for the terminally and critically ill based on the constitutional rights of the patients. Had the New York court decided its cases in terms of a constitutional analysis, it would have inhibited legislative action, since a legislature must respect constitutional rights.

The Massachusetts courts held that a person has a constitutional right to decline medical treatment but that judicial approval is required before treatment can be discontinued, except in a few circumstances such as orders not to resuscitate.[10] The New York court, by basing its decision on nonconstitutional grounds, held that when there was something similar to a living will declaring the person's intentions, judicial approval of nontreatment was not required.

The New Jersey case was the celebrated Karen Ann Quinlan case, in which the court asserted that the patient had a constitutional right to decline treatment.[11] The New Jersey court, however, required the approval of a hospital committee before granting the physicians and the hospital immunity from civil or criminal actions arising out of their actions.

Viewed against the background of the New Jersey and Massachusetts cases, the New York court thought it had made considerable progress along two fronts: it had proposed an analysis that allowed courts to remove themselves from the process of decision-making in ordinary cases by suggesting that a living will provides a sufficient basis to allow termination of treatment; and it had provided a basis for legislative intervention in deciding issues of health care delivery for the terminally and critically ill patient. The attempt to move away from the Massachusetts position, thus allowing for possible legislative action, is a positive development. The court, however, failed to see that any legislative action would probably start with the concept of the living will or some form of prior declaration of intentions. Thus the legislatures would offer solutions no different from those of the court, since the New York court failed to highlight the importance of the institutional context of the decision.[12]

The court that started legal developments concerning the right to die in the Karen Ann Quinlan case has had a recent opportunity to reflect upon the subsequent opinions handed down by other courts in similar cases. The New Jersey court does adopt the posture of the New York court in calling for living wills and legislative action, thus modifying its earlier holding. There is a dawning awareness that the institutional context of the decision is significant, although this awareness does not provide the overall framework that I propose.

The Case of a Nursing Home Patient

In *In the Matter of Claire C. Conroy,*[13] the New Jersey court was faced with a conflict between Mrs. Conroy's nephew and legal guardian, on the one hand, and her attending physician and the administrator of the nursing home where she lived, on the other. The nephew wanted the nasogastric feeding tube removed, whereas the physician and the administrator, a registered nurse, felt the tube should remain. Although the court noted that the nursing home, as an organization (i.e., its board of directors), took no position on whether the feeding tube should be removed, it did not attach any significance to this fact.[14]

In 1979, at the age of eighty, Claire Conroy was found to be incompetent; her only surviving relative, a nephew, was appointed her legal guardian. She suffered from what the court called "an organic brain syndrome"; this probably means that her neurological functioning was beginning to deteriorate from old age. The symptoms of this deterioration were manifested in periods of confusion.[15]

Apparently this confusion was sufficient in the nephew's view to require nursing home care. I say "apparently" because the court does not discuss the reasons for commitment to the nursing home, since it is supposedly irrelevant to its analysis. (Nevertheless, it will be shown later that the function of nursing homes is implicit in the court's guidelines.)[16] The court opinion does state that, upon her admission, Mrs. Conroy was fully mobile, able to follow directions, and in good physical condition even though she was confused about some things. Going into the nursing home was a significant event in her life, since on her nephew's own testimony, "all [Claire Conroy and her deceased sisters] wanted was to have her bills paid and *die in their own house.*"[17]

In Claire Conroy's case, admission to the nursing home must have been the most traumatic event of her adult life. She had lived in the same house since her childhood, never married, had few friends, and had been very close to her three sisters, all of whom had died. She had worked at the same company from her teenage years until retirement in her early sixties. Sometime after her admission to the nursing home, the court opinion states that she became "increasingly confused, disoriented, and physically dependent."[18]

While a resident of the nursing home, Conroy had one relatively short period of hospitalization for dehydration and a urinary tract infection in 1979. In 1982 she was hospitalized again for nearly three months because of a high temperature and dehydration. Early in this hospitalization, her physician from the nursing home noticed that she was not eating adequately and inserted a nasogastric tube that allowed medicine and nourishment to be administered. She was discharged from the hospital to the nursing home in November of 1982 with the tube left in place. In January, the tube was removed to make a second attempt to feed her by mouth; however, her ability to swallow had become so impaired that the tube was reinserted. Shortly afterward, her nephew, as legal guardian, brought a lawsuit to compel the treating physicians to remove the tube. The nursing home, as an organization, followed the physician's orders but was essentially neutral in that it would not oppose any order entered by the court.[19] By this time, Claire Conroy had become bedridden in a semifetal position, although she could move her head, neck, hands, and arms to a limited degree. She had several other medical complications, such as a gangrenous leg, but there was no specific life-threatening illness. She was now severely demented and unable to respond to verbal stimuli, although she responded to some external stimuli in a limited manner.

The basic contention of the nephew was that his aunt would have wanted the nasogastric tube removed because she "would not have allowed [it] to be inserted in the first place." He had refused to allow her gangrenous leg to be amputated during her most recent hospitalization because he claimed that she would have refused the amputation as well. He presented as evidence the fact that his aunt feared and avoided doctors. To his knowledge, she had never visited a doctor until she became incompetent.[20] When it became evident that she would never regain cognitive functioning, his view was that she would have preferred a "death with dignity" to a life maintained solely by machines.

The New Jersey Supreme Court accepted the nephew's view in formulating the issue as one of "What did the patient want?" For this purpose, the court assumed that the patient was competent and able to communicate. Yet it went on to develop an elaborate method of determining what the patient wanted when he or she was, in fact, unable to speak, which the record in Conroy's case did not meet. The court reviewed many previous opinions but was most impressed with the idea that individuals ought to express their wishes beforehand in a manner formal enough to be accepted by law; thus, the living will was seen as the best kind of evidence.[21]

Having developed an analysis that protects the rights of those who are mentally competent "to die of natural causes without medical intervention,"[22] the court went on to develop its legal analysis for incompetents such as Claire Conroy. Relying in part on the analysis developed by the New York courts, the court advised that a patient's intention to decline lifesaving treatment could be effectively stated in a living will, even in the absence of legislative action giving these documents legal effect. The court categorized this test as a purely subjective analysis.[23] There are many persons, such as Claire Conroy, who have not clearly expressed any prior intention, so the court felt compelled to develop legal tests that would allow the withdrawal of treatment. Under the state's power to supervise the care of wards by allowing the guardian to do what was in the "best interests" of the incompetent, the court devised two ways of determining that interest.

The first was called the "limited objective test" and required clear evidence of the patient's intentions to refuse treatment under circumstances based upon "medical evidence that burdens of treatment in terms of pain and suffering outweigh the benefits that the patient is experiencing."[24] In developing this test, the court indicated that it wanted a procedure to cover a situation where the evidence was less than conclusive, as, for instance, in a situation in which a general or vague living will did not meet the particular circumstances.

The second of these tests of a patient's best interests was called the "pure objective test." Under this test the court required a finding of net burdens over benefits and a further finding that the "recurring, unavoidable and severe pain of the patient's life with the treatment" is such that continued administration of the treatment would be inhumane.[25] The court asserted, without convincing proof in my opinion, that the evaluation of the patient's life in terms of pain or suffering still does not authorize the decision-maker to withdraw life-sustaining treatment based on his or her judgment about the

social worth of the patient's life.[26] Although an elaborate set of rules
was developed for determining the intentions of a person who cannot
speak, the court made clear that its ruling applies only to residents
in nursing homes.[27]

In accordance with traditional analysis, the court had to decide
upon procedures, such as who precisely could administer the various
tests of the patient's intentions. Here the court explicitly recognized
that procedures developed in the Quinlan case might be appropriate
for patients with certain medical conditions, but not for those like
Claire Conroy who are confined to nursing homes.[28] While pointing
out some obvious differences between nursing homes and hospitals,
the court noted that the New Jersey state legislature had passed
statutes attempting to deal with the variation of nursing homes from
the ideal. In the court's view, the decision for terminating any life-
sustaining treatment for nursing home patients should not conflict
with a statute designed to prevent the "abuse of rights" of nursing
home residents.

As a substantive matter, the court determined that the termination
of life-sustaining treatment for nursing home patients would not be
a "willful deprivation of services necessary to maintain a person's
physical and mental health," because the withdrawal or withholding
of treatment would be done to alleviate the patient's "pain."[29] This
determination is perhaps more important to the court's ruling than
is at first apparent, since a contrary ruling on this issue would have
terminated the case, with the court ruling that the legislature must
devise specific means for terminating care. But the court really could
not do this, having already built a constitutional limitation in *Quinlan.* The court then laid out the elaborate procedures that must be
followed.

First, the court imposed a legal prerequisite to substitute decision-
making in that there must be a legal finding of incompetence and the
appointment of a guardian. This finding is not in and of itself sufficient, since the court demands medical evidence that the person
lacks, and is not likely to regain, the capacity to make medical
decisions. Presumably, this requires evidence from a neurologist or
in some cases a psychiatrist. Second, with the court having established incompetence, any of the three tests for determining intention
could be used, provided the procedures that involved the notification
and participation of the Office of the Ombudsman for the Institutionalized Elderly were followed.

Once notified of the proposed termination of treatment of a nursing home patient, the ombudsman should regard such a proposal as
a possible abuse of the patient's rights, which would require an

investigation. The court then recommended that the ombudsman use discretionary powers to appoint two physicians not associated with the nursing home to confirm the diagnosis of the attending physician and nurses. If the medical prognosis and all other evidence, including available evidence about the patient's wishes, is in accordance, the guardian may withhold the life-supporting devices or treatments under any of the tests proposed by the court.

To make its legal opinion about nursing home patients consistent with its opinion in *Quinlan,* which concerned hospital-based patients, the court held that the participants would be immune from civil liability. But the court noted one difference: the ombudsman could still refer cases to the county prosecutor for criminal proceedings. Thus the guardians and the attending physician must convince the ombudsman of the correctness of their decision to withdraw treatment. Or, put in terms of the statute, there must be enough evidence to overcome the initial presumption that the withdrawal of life-sustaining treatment constitutes an abuse of the patient's rights.[30] This set of procedures meant, in the court's view, that there would be limited judicial involvement in the decisions to terminate treatment of nursing home patients. The court also felt it had left the area open to legislative intervention, since it had decided the case on common law rather than constitutional grounds.

It remained for the court to find whether the decision to terminate treatment in Claire Conroy's case was legally correct under its various tests. Despite what newspaper accounts may have indicated, the court found that the lower court was incorrect in ordering the feeding tube removed from Conroy,[31] and that the intermediate court was incorrect in its holding that the removal of the feeding tube would constitute homicide. Rather, the court administered its own tests and found the evidence insufficient. The court pointed out that there was no evidence of Claire Conroy's religious and moral beliefs, nor was there conclusive evidence that she was in extreme pain. With a general admonition to guardians and courts to be cautious, the court invited the legislature to deal with the many areas not addressed in the court's opinion concerning nursing home residents. Claire Conroy had died before the highest court decided the case, so there was no need to remand it.

Two salient features of the court's opinions are in need of detailed attention to demonstrate that an institutional approach would have better illuminated the underlying moral issues. First, the entire opinion is colored by a preoccupation with eliminating the amount of "pain" the patient is experiencing, confusing that with the apparent goal of promoting "death with dignity" in the face of modern medical technology. After presenting the facts of the case, the court stated:

> As scientific advances make it possible for us to live longer than ever before, even when our physical and mental capacities have been irrevocably lost, patients and their families are increasingly asserting a right to die a natural death without undue dependence upon medical technology or unnecessarily protracted agony—in short, a right to "die with dignity."[32]

As the dissenting justice pointed out, the two tests for determining "best interests" heavily depend on determining the amount of pain the patient is experiencing and would be likely to experience by further treatment.[33] It is important to recognize the court's assumption that "pain" is an objective factor that can be determined by a medical specialist.

Without presenting a discourse on the epistemology of pain, we should view pain in the context of serious illness as a sociopsychological phenomenon. We are most likely to confuse our own imagined pain (at seeing a debilitated woman of eighty-four) with the pain she is actually experiencing. Although this confusion of "self" and "other" has many beneficial features, it is possible for our wish that the supposed pain of the other would go away to be confused with a wish that the patient would die.[34] The trial judge in a rare moment of troubled candor demonstrated what our assumption about pain can do when he wrote:

> I think it is fair to say that everyone involved in this case wishes that this poor woman would die. This wish does not flow from any lack of concern for Claire Conroy. On the contrary, it flows from a very deep sympathy for her sad plight.[35]

The highest court did not deal explicitly with this statement except to disavow the quality-of-life implications of the trial judge's opinion. Instead, the court tried to objectify the matter of pain. In so doing, the highest court did not note what the institutional situation of Claire Conroy says about society's inability to deal with the problem of aging and prolonged death. This issue could have been addressed had the court openly explored the function of nursing homes.

The court could have addressed the institutional situation by inviting the nursing home involved to become an official party to the lawsuit. In this way, the court would have been asking for a functional differentiation of the roles of hospitals, nursing homes, and hospices. Such an extended analysis would clarify the evolving institution of the hospice.

Second, the New Jersey court, like the New York court, calls for legislative action but has invited the legislature only to make living wills or their functional equivalent legitimate. It is curious that the court did not interpret the New Jersey statute on nursing homes as inconsistent with its elaborate set of rules for terminating treatment. Had the New Jersey court been more critical in its evaluation of the statute's meaning, it would have seen that its opinion is built upon the assumption that law must provide a way of terminating life-sustaining treatment of nursing home patients in cases such as Claire Conroy's.

When the court examined the statutes covering the "rights" of such patients, it never occurred to it that the legislature had, in fact, dealt with this precise issue through deliberate inaction. In declaring that "it is the public policy of this State to secure for elderly patients, residents and clients of health care facilities [later defined to include nursing homes], serving their specialized needs and problems, the same civil and human rights guaranteed to all citizens,"[36] the court could have assumed that the legislature would have dealt with the important question of whether elderly patients in nursing homes should have the legal right to make living wills. If we assume that the overall purpose of these reform bills would include a section that gave patients the "right to die with dignity," we would simply be admitting that public discussion of the functions of the nursing home has skewed the major issue of whether dispensing death ought to be viewed as morally acceptable in the nursing home context. The failure of the legislature to have a section dealing with the issue of living wills meant the court was left with two options. It could have assumed that the legislature simply ignored this issue and left it to courts to develop the doctrines determining the withdrawal of treatment, which was essentially the position chosen by the court. The other option would have been to read into the statute a legislative unwillingness to authorize the removal of feeding tubes and other life-sustaining devices, either on the assumption that current practice was appropriate or that explicit legalization of the practice of terminating life support would be inappropriate in the nursing home context.

Had the court chosen the latter option, it would have had to move to constitutional grounds to reach its results, or it might have realized that its entire orientation was directed toward writing an opinion that gave guidelines concerning the withholding or termination of treatment. The court never considered the creative possibility of writing a less than definitive opinion. Such an approach would have led to an affirmation of the appellate court's decision not to allow the withdrawal of treatment. The court then could have announced a need to modify its approach, particularly its constitutional analysis in *Quinlan,* and its insistence on the necessity of immunity from subsequent judicial review. Ultimately the court failed to realize that its interaction with medicine had forced it to take on new roles in adjudication, roles that need to be clearly articulated.

The court's analysis points down one legislative path: legitimate the individual's supposed intentions about declining treatment; that is, make living wills somehow legally binding. The difficulty with the living will is conceptual, rather than procedural. The living will reflects a growing fear of social isolation that manifests itself in attempts to control unforeseeable events and a denial that debilitating illness would change our view of the world. The latter view is a reflection of the heroic notion of modern medicine in its least modest posture. Under this vision, for instance, there is a certainty that a cure for cancer will be found, that artificial organs will be perfected, and that biochemical interventions will somehow arrest the aging process. Those who accept this heroic vision often suffer the most disillusionment when they discover uncertainty or doubt within medicine. This reaction also leads to an antitechnological bias that postulates the existence of a "natural death" as something morally superior to the death suffered by such patients as Claire Conroy.

These disillusioned people, in which I include the court in the Conroy case, hold a romantic notion of medical professionals as healers which fails to integrate the enormous insights and progress of modern medicine. Two examples from the opinion illustrate this romanticizing of the role of healer. First, in its discussion of maintaining the integrity of the medical profession, the New Jersey court quotes Francis Bacon on the role of the physician in regard to withholding treatment. The court stated:

> Medical ethics do not require medical intervention in disease at all costs. As long ago as 1624, Francis Bacon wrote, "I esteem it the office of a physician not only to restore health, but to mitigate pain and dolours; not only when such mitigation may conduce a recovery, but when it may serve to make a fair and easy passage."[37]

The biochemical and technological tools available to the physician of Bacon's day were primitive in comparison to those available to the modern physician. Bacon's statement, for example, when applied to a physician of his day faced with pneumonia, meant that the physician had to watch the disease take its natural course. A modern physician would expect the patient to be cured with a variety of modern drugs. The court does not imply that such biomedical intervention is generally bad, only that such intervention may not be appropriate in cases of patients who are terminally ill or in a persistent vegetative state. The court fails to acknowledge, however, that

Francis Bacon and the modern physician live in two wholly different cultural contexts. Statements made in one cultural context do not have the same significance in another. And even if these statements are treated as principles of the physician's role, we should recognize that changing roles mean those principles have different implications.

The second illustration from the court's opinion is the court's view of Claire Conroy's attending physician. On the one hand, the court treated him as simply another witness rather than a potential litigant to the lawsuit. It noted, for instance, that the attending physician stated that the removal of the tube would not be in accordance with acceptable medical practice, but failed to attribute any legal significance to this position. The court explained his position as simply "She's a human being, and I guess she has a right to live if it's possible."[38] This is an inadequate presentation of the physician's moral position. Had the court given his moral position greater credence by identifying it with the traditional notion that the physician is to be with his patient at the moment of death or considering it as contrary to the Hippocratic injunction to do no harm, it could not have been dismissed without discussion.

On the other hand, the court projects a subtle criticism of the attending physician. It suggested that his once-a-month visits provided a definite example of the lack of sufficient medical attention to elderly nursing home patients.[39] Yet a few paragraphs later, the court admits that medical decisions for nursing home patients are clearly more foreseeable than those reached in hospitals. The lack of acute medical problems would seem to justify less attention on the part of the physician once major decisions about the course of the patient's medical condition have been established. Why then is the court critical of the attending physician? The only explanation is that the court either finds his opinion embarrassing or identifies him with the medical professionals who are depriving elderly patients of a "death with dignity."

Commitment to a nursing home implies that other social institutions, most notably the family, are unable to cope with elderly members of society. In Claire Conroy's case it is worth questioning why we assume that a person who has lost some functioning needs this type of institutional care. The social and financial means to support her in her home as her condition simply deteriorates may not be available, but there are social options other than the nursing home that we have not yet explored.

By admitting that there are other options to nursing home care, the court could deal with the function of hospice care as one way of distinguishing between the terminally ill and the critically ill. Many nursing home residents are not terminally ill when admitted, and some, like Conroy, do not even fit the category of critically ill. Her case demonstrates how easily we assume that a critically ill person is a terminally ill patient. A refusal to treat her as terminally ill would be a social affirmation of the sanctity of human life in the face of modern medicine. As a body deteriorates, we should not assume that there is a loss of human dignity.

The way in which individuals die does have a great deal to do with the social fabric of a society. In a world with modern medicine we have become anxious for a "quick death" and a "painless death." Unless we build a social structure for dealing with those anxieties, we run the risk of inflicting death on others in order to protect ourselves from our own anxiety. An institutional approach that focuses on the function of the nursing home is one way in which law can help contribute to the building of such a social structure.

An institutional approach would have affirmed the intermediate appellate court's ruling that it was legally impermissible to remove the feeding tube from Claire Conroy. Such an affirmation is necessary to establish the presumption in favor of sustaining life in the absence of a social consensus that there is no "life" to sustain. In Claire Conroy's case, there was an obvious lack of consensus since the primary caregivers, the attending physician and the nurse administrator, opposed the removal of the feeding tube on the theory that this opposition is what the patient would have wanted.

The New Jersey court developed an analysis that assumed that the individual patient is the source of moral wisdom and certainty. The court ignored an opportunity to deal with the Claire Conroy case from an institutional perspective, which would have insisted on participation by the nursing home in any such lawsuit. Since Claire Conroy was already dead by the time the case reached the highest court, the court could have pointed out that the nursing home was responsible for developing a plan to ensure that termination of treatment is done in a morally acceptable fashion. The court could then have suggested that it, along with the legislature, would review this plan. Unless the court articulates the function of the nursing home, it is likely to be seen as simply an adjunct to the modern hospital. But it is important to realize that commitment to a nursing home has broad social implications about the nature of "family" and its limited capacity to care in the face of the disabilities of age.

Conclusion

Although the study of how society confronts death is a fundamental feature of any given social structure, the institutional approach does not propose that medicine's social function is to wage a battle against mortality.[40] Rather, the institutional approach suggests that medicine's function is to provide care and law's function is to provide a structure that allows for the evolution of society's concepts of death, life, and health. The effect of the institutional approach can be illustrated by two points made in the earlier analysis of the case involving the removal of feeding tubes from nursing home residents.

First, law should not assume that a nursing home is simply another hospital. The nursing home is a discrete institution whose functions must be distinguished from those of general hospitals, hospices, and facilities for the mentally retarded. In the context of a society with an increasingly aging population, the nursing home's function must be defined in terms of the realistic capacity for caretaking of relatives and friends. Law can encourage such a functional definition by urging nursing homes to develop policies on feeding tubes and on the level of medical care that will be provided. Not all nursing homes need to have the same policy on these matters, but there must be written policies that families, friends, physicians, and potential nursing home residents can read and discuss before making the fundamental shift in social relationships that life in a nursing home represents.

Second, the institutional approach rejects the notion that the imagined will of the nursing home resident or any critically ill patient is the ultimate source of moral authority for a course of action. Rather, the critically ill person is entitled to care, whether or not medical intervention is involved. In emphasizing the role of caring, we would come to understand that caring means social connections. It may also mean sharing the suffering, the pain, the ambivalence, the anger, and often the silence of a person who is critically ill.

The judiciary has generally acknowledged that its analysis of the morally complex question of death and dying would be resolved in a better manner if legislatures took action. In particular, courts have suggested that some type of living will is appropriate and have allowed for more legislative flexibility by basing more recent decisions on nonconstitutional grounds. But the living will, from an institutional perspective, is an inadequate conceptual framework for law's handling of these moral issues. The living-will approach assumes that one individual—the patient—is the sole arbiter of the meaning of death, when we know that death is not only a deeply personal experience but a profoundly social one as well.

Chapter 5

Legislative Reform
and the Question of Dying

Hospitals, as organizations, should be encouraged to assume responsibility for developing methods of treating the critically ill—the modern problem of caring. We need an overall legal approach that will encourage medicine to concern itself not only with restoring health but also with allowing death to take place in a morally acceptable way. We have to consider whether the ethos of modern medicine provides all participants—from the patient and his or her family to the medical establishment—with an understanding of the "rite of passage." We need law to support a program ancillary to the hospital or even distinctly separate, the hospice, which has as its chief function the care of the terminally ill.

Much of the criticism directed at judicial intervention in medicine is based on the theory that legislatures are better equipped to deal with the moral issues raised by modern medicine. Presumably, legislative action provides more certainty than judicial opinions. Such criticism does not realize that legal interaction with medicine is forcing a transformation of the judicial process. More importantly, such criticism fails to acknowledge that legislative reforms to date have adopted the same highly individualistic approach exhibited by judges in dealing with the issues of terminating care.

"Natural" Death and Moral Consensus

California provides a good illustration of the implicit need for additional work in this area. The state legislature has enacted several pieces of legislation in response to judicial activity in cases involving the termination of treatment. California also witnessed the first modern attempt to prosecute physicians for decisions to terminate treatment.

Shortly after the *Quinlan* case was decided, the California legislature enacted the Natural Death Act. This act sought to affirm the legal right of individuals to put a stop to life-sustaining measures by establishing a procedure that provided for written directives to physicians for the termination of treatment.[1] This statute gave legal validity to the living will, although the legislature wisely did not call its statute the Living Will Act. The statute also adopted the existing perspective of law by sanctifying the doctor-patient relationship, since the directive is to the physician rather than to a spouse, friend, or other family member. This legal supervision of the doctor-patient relationship is given moral justification by suggesting that the death experienced by the writer of a directive is a "natural" death as distinct from the artificial prolongation of life.

Nevertheless, there are both conceptual difficulties—social and medical—and practical difficulties with this statute. On the conceptual level, the statute assumes that there is a point at which death is "natural" and that this point can be determined objectively by a modern physician. A "life-sustaining procedure," for instance, is defined in the statute as any "mechanical or other artificial means," the use of which would only "artificially prolong the moment of death and where, in the judgment of the attending physician, death is imminent whether or not such procedures are utilized."[2]

This assumption, that there is an objectively determined point of natural death, is curious from a social and medical perspective. From a social perspective, death remains a personal phenomenon. For those witnessing a person dying, that experience is interpreted according to personal religious and philosophical views. Even advocates of new legislative definitions of death recognize its uniquely personal character and thus allow for a form of personalization in the declaration of death.[3]

From a medical perspective, even the newer definitions of brain death are subject to modification in light of the growth of scientific knowledge. A definition of brain death proposed less than twenty years ago has as part of its legal definition the general phrase "prevailing medical standards" rather than a delimiting list of tests. Allowing for the growth of knowledge in its continually evolving definition of death, society progressively cuts down the risk of error in determining brain death. As a result, our notion of a "natural" death constantly changes.

On the more practical level, however, the individualistic approach of the California statute fails to recognize that death increasingly takes place in the organizational context of a hospital or nursing home. This means that the doctor and the patient are not isolated but surrounded by many others who might also share the experience. As a result, family members and nurses attending the patient may have different views about the impending death and appropriate moral action.

A simple example illustrates the practical difficulty of implementing the legislature's individualistic approach. Suppose that a California man in his late fifties who has signed a directive as authorized by the statute becomes critically ill. Furthermore, suppose he has been the victim of an automobile accident and sustained numerous injuries that have left him in a coma from which the physicians do not expect him to recover. In this sense, he suffers from what the California statute calls a "terminal condition."[4] Assume that his condition is such that he is able to breathe without the assistance of a respirator but needs intravenous intake to supply food and antibiotics against infection. Assume further that the critically ill patient has previously signed the directive after discussions with his physician and his lawyer, but without the knowledge of his wife. The first time the wife of the patient becomes aware of his "wishes" is when the physician reports that her husband is not expected to recover from the coma and that, in accordance with his written directive, the feeding tubes will be removed, leading to his death within a few days. The wife immediately objects, indicating that she had no prior knowledge about the written directive.

Does the physician have the moral right to attempt to ensure that the patient dies a "natural death" despite the wife's vehement objection? The answer is no, for the fundamental reason that the patient's wife is presumably the human being most emotionally involved with the patient. The presumption stands that the wife has the greatest social claim on determining her husband's outcome. Following his death, she will have to cope with the social, economic, and emotional consequences of their life together in relief, grief, or simple disillusionment. Here we understand the full implication of the assertion that death is a social phenomenon.

What happens now? The physician can take the same course as that taken in the absence of any written directive—with what Robert Burt calls "a silent patient"[5]—engage the wife, other family members, and those involved in the patient's care in a dialogue about what course to follow. During those conversations, the physician is entitled to give not only a medical prognosis but also the information received from the patient in the form of the directive. But the written directive signed by the patient does not give the physician the moral right to act without considering the total social context.

The social context may be confused, of course, by conflicting feelings about the removal of the feeding tubes and the wife's pain in dealing with her husband's critical illness and impending death. Under such uncertainty physicians are likely to assert that the California legislature has relieved them of the responsibility of dealing with ethical and moral confusion by putting the physician under a legal requirement to follow the wishes of the patient. Or, stated in even stronger terms, whatever the uncertainties about the physician's moral duty, the legislature has made it a legal duty to carry out the wishes of the patient—in this case, to remove the feeding apparatus over the objection of his wife.

Does the California Natural Death Act in fact compel the physician to carry out the wishes of the patient in face of the objections of a family member? Would a lawyer advise the physician in California to remove the feeding tube in the face of the spouse's objection? Taking the question in either of its forms, the answer is no for a number of reasons. In its judgment about the rights of individuals to refuse life-sustaining treatment, the legislature did not establish a coercive mechanism for carrying out the patient's directive. In the normal case, in which the individual has signed the directive before having a terminal condition, the statute specifically states that there is no criminal or civil liability for *failing* to carry out the directive.[6] Rather, the statute implies that the physician is guilty only of unprofessional conduct if he or she fails to carry out the directive and then fails to take steps to transfer the patient to a physician who will do so.

What this provision means is that if the physician has any qualms about carrying out the directive, he or she can refrain from doing so without fear of a lawsuit from the patient's estate. Furthermore, because of another provision, the physician could even carry out the directive without fear of a lawsuit from the wife, having been granted immunity from civil and criminal prosecution.[7] Any objections become relevant only if the physician treats them as relevant. In some cases, if the physician thought a spouse's objection should morally prevent the removal of the feeding tubes, the physician is required under the statute to attempt to find a physician willing to carry out the directive despite the spouse's objection.[8] The statute deals explicitly with the physician's own moral claims but treats the objections of others as legally insignificant.

As a result, the California statute leaves the difficult moral decisions to the discretion of the physician rather than offering a moral consensus. The moral consensus hoped for is difficult to achieve because death is no longer a home-centered event and is likely to take place in the hospital or the nursing home.

Not surprisingly, the California legislature recognized a few years later that providing a clear mechanism by which a person could appoint someone else to make health care decisions in the event of incompetency dealt more directly with the social reality of dying

than the Natural Death Act. The Durable Power of Attorney Act
allows individuals to appoint someone to make health care decisions
in the event of their disability. While a person, before becoming a
patient, could appoint someone else to act as agent for health care
decisions, the statute recognizes the uncertainties of social life and
our attitudes about death. For instance, it is clear that despite the
formalistic legal document appointing the agent, a physician is to
treat the oral statement of the patient revoking the appointment as
binding upon the physician and to note the revocation in the patient's
medical record. Furthermore, the statute deals specifically with the
family situation by its implicit recognition that normally among
married persons the spouse would be the agent for health care decisions.[9]

Despite this greater degree of recognition of the social context of
death, the legislature has provided for a total notion of substitute
decision-making. First, there are some health care decisions that
cannot be authorized by an agent, even if the written document
making the appointment purports to give the agent this power. These
decisions are commitment to a mental hospital, convulsive treatment, psychosurgery, sterilization, and abortion.[10] These exclusions
recognize that a host of other values related to health cannot be
appropriately resolved by the social mechanism of appointing an
agent. Second, the legislature noted one situation where the physician or other health care provider should retain the discretion to
ignore a clear directive of the agent: if the agent authorizes the
withdrawal of a treatment necessary to keep the patient, the principal, alive, the health care professional cannot be subject to criminal
or civil proceedings or professional disciplinary actions for failing to
execute the agent's directive.[11] As to the issue of death, the physician
or health professional maintains ultimate authority to determine
whether to dispense death because of the fundamental institutional
context of modern medicine.

Thus a moral consensus about the appropriate point to stop or
withhold treatment must be found in the institutional context in
which death occurs, not in the abstract dyads of physician-patient or
physician-agent. A legislative approach that saw death in an institutional context might pass a statute ensuring the right of patients to
die in their own homes. Such a statute is not likely to be enacted, nor
am I suggesting that it is a wise policy. But thinking about the alleged
"right to die with dignity" or "right to die a natural death" in terms
of establishing a legal framework for returning the experience of
dying to the home highlights some of society's ambivalence about
death in this modern scientific age. Most families are not psychologically equipped to deal with a home-centered death. Perhaps our faith

in the progress of modern medicine has led to a general inability to cope with death, with the result that the family needs the social support of modern medicine. This does not mean the techniques of modern medicine must always be used, only that the decisions about care of critically ill patients must be made in the modern medical context. This means having access to the medical establishment in the decision-making process.

The legislature, in its analysis of the concept of "death with dignity," ought to have enacted a legal framework that allows for the growth of hospice care, either as an adjunct to hospitals or as a separate institution. As an institution, the hospice must recognize the rites of passage, the crucial relationship between appropriate care and death. The concept of rites of passage is important because the ethos of modern medicine is to encourage us to equate all forms of caring with treatment that preserves life. Some context is needed to make all participants in the drama of death, including physicians and nurses, aware that the goal has switched from preserving life to caring in the face of impending death.

The hospice has become an important institution because it provides a social context in which it can be morally acceptable to allow death to occur. As the hospice movement has developed in the United States,[12] the most important social function it provides is support for both patient and family. Moreover, a decision to move to hospice care does not mean a totally antimodern technological bias, since some aspects of modern medical establishment can be part of hospice care. For instance, in the context of hospice care, what might be deemed socially and medically inappropriate in other contexts—such as the administration of heroin as a painkiller—could be morally "correct."[13]

Consideration of hospice care would require the legislature to examine the reasons that have so far inhibited the growth of this evolving institution. Modern medicine has looked primarily to the hospital for its mode of organization, and the legislature may find that many laws and regulations prevent or severely limit the growth of hospice care. Such a long-range examination would help the legislature to recognize the institutional context of modern medicine.

Should Criminal Prosecution Be Authorized?

Even in California, the institutional context would not provide a panacea for solving certain moral problems, because limitations on a doctor's or other health provider's course of action in allowing death have not been determined. This lack of legal and moral guidelines is nowhere more apparent than in recent attempts in California to criminally prosecute several physicians for removing a life-supporting apparatus from a critically ill patient. The various opinions by the judges who reviewed the evidence are significant because they bear upon recent legislative action.

The patient whose death was the source of the attempted criminal prosecution, Clarence Herbert, suffered cardiac arrest following a surgical operation. Although his heartbeat was restored, he lapsed into a coma. After three days, it was determined that he had suffered severe brain damage that left him in a vegetative state. The medical experts involved apparently predicted that his vegetative state was permanent ("apparently," because at this stage of the proceedings none of the physicians involved chose to testify at the hearing before the magistrate).

What the attending physician told the patient's family is unclear, but the patient's wife and his eight children all signed a written request that read:

> We the family of Clarence LeRoy Herbert on this day of August 29, 1982, would like all machines taken off that are sustaining life. We release all liability to hospital, doctor, and staff. The Family.[14]

The wife testified that she was told that her husband was "brain dead."[15] The pathological reports, however, indicated that the patient was not brain dead by prevailing medical standards but that he had suffered severe brain damage.

The attending physician ordered the intravenous feeding tubes removed, after receiving the signed statement from the family. About a week after removal of the feeding tube and the moisturizing collar, the patient died of several causes, the principal one being a deficiency of oxygen to the brain.[16]

Without reviewing all the testimony presented to the magistrate, we can address significant conflicts in the evidence. First, a conflict arose between the patient's wife and some of the nurses concerning who first suggested that the food support system be removed.[17] Second, there was conflict between family members and the hospital staff as to the level of care to be given to the patient after the food support systems had been removed. The family objected to certain routine procedures with comatose patients, such as turning to prevent bedsores, because they did not want him to be disturbed.[18] The reasons for this conflict were not explored in any of the opinions, but the wife did testify she did not think it was appropriate to "feed a dead man." If she were under the impression that her husband was brain dead, it is possible to understand her reluctance to have him fed.

For the moment, I shall ignore the legal analysis of the magistrate, whose opinion dismissing the indictment was reviewed by the trial judge. Instead, I shall concentrate on differences in the approaches of the trial judge, who held the indictment was legally sufficient to allow the case to be presented to a jury, and the intermediate appellate court, which dismissed the indictment and called for legislative action.[19]

The trial judge's opinion presents a concise analysis of the legal issues regarding the charges of murder and conspiracy to commit murder that had been brought against two of the doctors involved in Mr. Herbert's case. The trial judge's duty is to state the basic elements of the crime charged. He noted without discussion that the litigants had not cited any legal authority defining the physician's duty to the patient, but he asserted that the legal duty encompassed sustaining the patient's life. From his reading of California law, the judge determined that the failure of a person to perform this legal duty could be the basis of a homicide prosecution. Then, without questioning the many specific findings of "fact" by the magistrate, the trial judge sought to interpret those facts in light of the legal standard for a homicide prosecution. Under this straightforward analysis, it was apparent that the actions of the physicians in removing the feeding support systems and the moisturizing devices shortened the patient's life. It only remained to determine if the shortening was done in an unlawful manner.

The trial judge looked to existing law to answer the question, which would also determine whether a jury could hear the full evidence. Is there something in law that would clearly make the removal of the life-sustaining apparatus lawful? His answer was no, for two reasons, both having to do with recent legislative enactments.

The first of these legislative enactments was the California Natural Death Act. Since the patient had not signed a directive or a living will, the judge reasoned that immunity from criminal prosecution was not available to the physicians, even with the signed consent of his family.[20]

Furthermore, the trial judge noted a particular policy declaration in the Natural Death Act that instructed him how to construe the indictment. A section at the end stated:

> Nothing in this chapter shall be construed to condone, authorize, or approve mercy killing, or to permit any affirmative or deliberate act or omission to end life other than to permit the natural process of dying as provided in this chapter.[21]

Under this reading, the trial judge saw a clear legislative directive to allow criminal indictments of individuals who took steps to hasten the death of critically ill patients outside the framework provided by the statute.

The trial judge buttressed his interpretation of the Natural Death Act by considering whether the patient was legally dead at the time the feeding tubes were removed. He noted that California had enacted a statute requiring that there be irreversible cessation of either the circulatory and respiratory functions or all brain functions in order for a person to be considered legally dead. The facts, as found by the magistrate, did not conclusively establish that the patient's condition was irreversible, but only that he was in a state of deep coma.[22]

The trial judge treated the indictment as presumptively valid and then proceeded to define the elements of the crime. He asserted that there was a legal duty on the part of the physician to maintain life. He then looked to legislative enactments to see if that legal duty had been modified in light of modern developments in medicine. He read those legislative enactments narrowly rather than broadly and found that neither the recently enacted California Natural Death Act nor the Uniform Determination of Death Act removed the duty from the physician. He recognized that as the facts were developed at trial or as the jury interpreted the evidence, there might not be sufficient legal evidence for a finding of guilt. He emphasized that, at this stage of the proceedings, there need only be a "strong suspicion of guilt"[23] rather than proof beyond a reasonable doubt (required for an actual criminal conviction).

In contrast, the intermediate appellate court started with the assumption that traditional conceptions of criminal liability should *not* be used in the case. Near the beginning of its opinion, the court stated:

> [T]his issue must be determined against a background of legal and moral considerations which are of fairly recent vintage and which as a result *have not, in our opinion, been adequately addressed by the Legislature.* . . . [I]t appears to us that a murder prosecution is a poor way to design an ethical and moral code for doctors who are faced with decisions concerning the use of costly and extraordinary "life support" equipment.[24]

With this perspective, the court started its legal analysis with the California murder statute rather than with the common-law idea of the duty of the physician used by the trial judge. This is a significant difference in approach; it has long been recognized that "failure to act" as a basis of criminal liability has always presented unique problems for criminal jurisprudence.

Basing its analysis on the California murder statute, the court looked to determine whether there was sufficient evidence that the physicians "killed" the patient. The court opinion suggests that it is legally improper to indict physicians for murder unless there is evidence that they took active steps to end the patient's life. Under this analysis, the implicit threat is not withdrawal of life-support means in doubtful situations but what might be thought of as active euthanasia. The court's technical reasoning led it to the issue of determining whether the physicians' conduct was unlawful within the California homicide statutes. In answer, the court explicitly stated that principles other than those of criminal law must be used.

In looking to other California statutes, the court asserted that the legislature had dealt "partially" with the problems that had arisen because of modern medicine's ability to sustain life.[25] After criticizing the Natural Death Act for not being broader, the court read the statute as inconclusive because of a clause stating that the act did not change any other rights a person might have to terminate or forgo life-sustaining treatment.[26] The court reasoned that competent patients had the right to control the course of medical treatment. It then specifically held that the Natural Death Act does not constitute the only means of terminating life-support measures. Nor did the court find the statute on brain death as controlling as the trial judge had.

Only at this point did the court deal with the case in the same terms as those of the trial judge, by analyzing the duty of the physician to act under the circumstances of a comatose patient who has little chance of recovery. The court concluded that, as a matter of law, the physician had no legal or moral duty to continue treatment. In reaching its decision, the court relied on the reasoning in the *Saikewicz* and *Quinlan* cases to suggest that, once there is no benefit from a treatment, a physician does not have a clear duty to continue it, even if death is a certain consequence.[27] The court failed to note, however, that the statement of the physician's duty in those cases came from standards developed in malpractice litigation and not from an analysis of the function of criminal law, thus suggesting that malpractice law alone provides the limits of physician action.

In addition, the court established a form of immunity from criminal prosecution in its desire to provide physicians with what it called some "general guidelines" for future conduct.[28] The court went so far as to quote language from the *Quinlan* case in its attempt "to free physicians, in the pursuit of their healing vocation," holding that there were no possible circumstances under which physicians could be liable for murder. The role the court saw for the legislature was to deal with the procedural issues of whether courts and legally appointed guardians must be involved in the decision to terminate treatment when the patient has no reasonable chance of recovery.

Despite the court's assumption that its substantive decision about potential criminal liability needed no legislative review, I contend that the court's opinion raises questions of appropriate criminal law policy. A reader could infer from the opinion that alleged misjudgments to remove life-sustaining equipment can never be subject to a criminal homicide prosecution. This implication is dangerous because it ignores criminal law standards as the background against which the standards of civil liability operate. The difference between the functions of criminal and civil liability in medical issues needs to be explored.

The function of civil liability in the form of the malpractice system, as explained in chapter 1, is to allow medicine as an institution to be the primary allocator and distributor of health entitlements. Through an evolving series of legal decisions, law has established a framework of rules within which those allocations and distributions must take place. The function of criminal law is to provide legal sanctions against those health care providers who operate outside the rules.

With specific reference to the case before it, the California court should have seen that the death-dispensing function is not one that belongs solely to health care institutions and officials. Death is not, in the court's words, solely a medical matter; it is a social and personal phenomenon with profound implications for the way we see ourselves as related individuals within the cultural context of a given society. Because of its social importance, death is a phenomenon in which criminal law does play a role.

The lack of consensus about the appropriateness of the termination of life support should have made the court more cautious in its approach in Mr. Herbert's case. At the very least, some of the key participants in the death-dispensing process had either severe misunderstandings of the medical situation or profound moral qualms about the appropriateness of withdrawing life-sustaining treatment. If we think of criminal law as providing the background standard of the social duty of the physician, we can see the potential intervention of criminal law as ensuring that those with a social interest understand the meaning of the medical prognosis.

The court was probably correct in its view that the charge of murder was inappropriate in a situation in which, at worst, the physicians acted too hastily in withdrawing life support. But under traditional analysis, the court should have considered whether these actions constituted the lesser form of criminal homicide, manslaughter, the unlawful taking of life without the express or implied intent to injure the victim.[29]

The California legislature and other legislatures must review the role of criminal liability in the medical area. They should consider legislation that would establish manslaughter as the appropriate crime to charge when physicians make misjudgments concerning their death-dispensing functions. In the context of the evolving institutions of hospices and the unclear role of nursing homes in death situations, physicians must be given the ultimate responsibility of presenting options to the participants in the patient's death. By promulgating criminal standards, the legislatures would establish the social function of physicians.

Legislative consideration of criminal liability must necessarily encompass a review of the many cases alleging to establish the right to die, since it is now apparent that the two are linked in the minds of judges and of the public. In my view, the physician's potential criminal liability must be seen in the institutional context in which he or she operates. The legislature should reject the ideal of a living will as its starting point and think first of hospitals as large-scale organizations with the potential for some degree of social control.

Health care facilities need to accept responsibility for controlling the individual physician's decision by declining the invitation to write detailed procedural rules for decisions about terminally ill and critically ill patients. State legislatures could pass legislation that would prohibit orders for terminating or withholding treatment in the absence of approval of an appropriate hospital committee.[30] While this is an admittedly vague standard, such legislation would encourage hospitals and nursing homes to set up a variety of structures to review decisions that are likely to lead to a patient's death. It is important to point out that there is no interference with those discretionary decisions designed to preserve life or to provide healing, only those in which the physician becomes society's dispenser of death. Were a legislature to indicate that, without institutional approval, a physician would be guilty of manslaughter, the incentive would be to discover what structures would be appropriate. A hospital faced with such legislation would not have great difficulty in determining what kinds of committees are necessary. The perspective on the cases offered here provides some important guidelines.

First, the committees should not be "ethics committees," because the legislation implies that the ethical responsibility belongs to the attending physicians. Nor is the hospital or its professionals necessarily any more expert about the ethics of these situations than anyone else. The committees, consisting primarily of physicians, would be a means of confirming the medical prognosis based on the theory that there must be social assurance that the medical diagnosis is correct before termination can be undertaken. Thus, there might be different committees for "brain death," "persistent vegetative states," and the "severely defective newborn."

Second, the hospital's own bylaws or rules should require that the attending physician convene the committee in person, but only after informing the patient, if conscious, and any relatives, nurses, or other persons who have become participants in the patient's care. The function of the consultation requirement is to ensure that the physician has acknowledged his or her own professional responsibility vis-à-vis the patient and the community. A hospital bylaw of this sort further suggests that, from the hospital's perspective, the physician must be willing to take personal responsibility for the decision to terminate life. The physician cannot hide behind the collectivism of a committee. What is being suggested is a concept of professional responsibility within the context of the institution of medicine so that physicians start to think about issues of medical ethics in terms of their public role rather than in terms of their own values or personal preferences.[31]

One other legislative modification of existing case law is necessary for a viable institutional approach. The legislature must clearly state that neither health care institutions nor physicians can bring suit to compel treatment in terminally ill or critically ill cases. These suits simply prevent hospitals and physicians from proceeding when they cannot obtain consent, such as in *Storar*. Such a provision would prevent modern medical institutions from imposing their views of health upon individuals who are trying to cope with their own death or that of a loved one. Thus, when physicians feel a patient needs treatment, they would be forced to rely not upon the coercive powers of the law but upon their powers of persuasion and their growing capacity to be healers with technical and scientific skills.

This suggested legislative approach reflects my belief that the lack of social consensus about care for terminally ill and critically ill patients is a function of modern medicine itself. I would encourage legislatures to define the role of courts and hospitals as organizations that take account of the realities of modern medicine. They should, in addition, eschew legal analysis using "consent" as its moral foundation. The risk of the current approach of focusing exclusively on the doctor-patient relationship is twofold. Either law will be ignored because it fails to take account of the value system of modern medicine and inhibits the proper functioning, or, in our haste to find sure and quick answers to our societal quandary about hospital-centered deaths, we will begin to make decisions that undermine our reverence for life.

Conclusion

Legislatures must enact legislation that encourages the growth of hospices. Such legislation should also realize that building such an effective social institution to help with the rites of passage into death will take considerable time. Nor should the legislatures consider the hospice the answer to all questions about whether a person, particularly an elderly patient, is being killed or simply allowed to die.

Rather, in light of recent judicial opinions, legislatures must examine whether special legislation is needed to deal with the criminal liability of physicians and other health care professionals. The reformulation of the standards for criminal liability is a way of establishing the social function of medicine: When criminal sanctions are authorized, there is a clear concern about the proper social functioning of the physician. The exercise of control of physicians through potential criminal liability is of paramount importance in Western countries.

The institutional approach will help to make possible public debate about health care policy in this country. Once we abandon the individualistic perspective that places one life against another and move to the institutional approach, we can highlight issues that are clearly germane but often not considered in the current approach.

As long as we keep insisting on living wills in the context of an increasingly aging and cost-conscious society, we run the risk of encouraging individuals to sign their own death warrants as the only means of maintaining any form of social "responsibility." The challenge is to develop a structure that encourages caring in the face of all types of debilitating illnesses. We need to focus on the capacity for caring, rather than on "preserving life" or "death with dignity," as the ultimate test of the social fabric.

Chapter 6

Caring for Children

Children ideally live in families, which themselves exist for social-
izing the young. Families are essentially caregiving institutions in
which adults articulate through time those sets of private values that
give meaning to their lives. A central dilemma for us is: How do we
promote the family in terms of public policy when we have defined
it as intensively private? Now and in the future, beginning with
conception as an increasingly technological event, law must embrace
an expanded vision of caring for children.

A risk to a child's health and life is a catastrophic social event since
impairment or death severely fractures the sense of continuity
through time that children provide their parents. Law recognizes the
precarious position of children by declaring them legally incompetent and in need of the protection of others, as persons entitled to
custody rather than liberty. What law has done (or failed to do) to
resolve conflicts about the care of severely impaired newborns, abortion for teenagers, and cancer treatment for children understandably
invokes strong and often opposing feelings about what is the "caring" and "just" thing to do.

One possible response to these strong reactions is to suggest an
analysis that would provide a clear legal matrix of either "children's
rights" or "family autonomy." A children's rights analysis would see
law as the ultimate protection of the child's potential for autonomous
decision-making and then recognize a child's right to make certain
health care decisions, such as whether to abort a fetus, independent
of parental or other custodial interference. Parents and children are
linked within families: a child looks to an adult functioning as a
parent for nurture, guidance, and that set of private values that
defines continuity. These definitions are deliberately circular; one
cannot conceive of a child without postulating an adult who cares
for the child. The family autonomy approach would exclusively

delegate decision-making regarding health care decisions for children and parents to the individual family involved, on the theory that there is no more relevant social consensus of what is the morally correct thing to do. But both approaches ignore the uncertainty inherent in modern medicine. In addition, both approaches ignore the fact that lawsuits about health care for children are not only a manifestation of the uncertainty caused by rapid medical advances, but also the result of a fundamental misconception concerning the role of law and medicine in relationship to other institutions in society, such as the family.

Other caretaking institutions share with law and medicine a concern for the welfare of the child. If, as I suggest, we can avoid a totally rationalistic and scientific approach to health care decision-making for children, we would implicitly give those other caretaking institutions, such as the family, a voice in defining the "health" of the child. This chapter establishes a framework that defines the function of medicine, law, and other caretaking institutions in medical decision-making for children. In so doing, we must never accept the notion that medical or legal decisions can be separated from the social fabric in which the child lives.

First I shall discuss the social and moral implications of a parental decision to commit a child to a state mental hospital, to explain why we should start with the assumption that parents have authority to make such health care decisions. Second, I shall discuss a case involving whether conventional treatment for cancer can be legally refused for a child. Analysis of this case will provide an opportunity to demonstrate the inadequacy of the prevailing legal analysis of "substituted judgment" and its accompanying question of who should then make that judgment. The better question in terms of delineating moral problems is: Under which institutional perspective should we view the problem of cancer treatment for children? Third, I shall discuss a case of judicial authorization of a kidney transplant between identical twins where, in fact, there was no real conflict about the parental decision to proceed. In this instance, I shall demonstrate the limited efficacy of legal intervention in many health decisions for children, despite the uncertainty and moral confusion that are often involved. Finally, I examine two cases without immediate life-and-death consequences—abortion for a minor and a heart operation for a mentally retarded child—to demonstrate that families are the primary custodians of a child's health.

The legal perspective I propose takes full account of the irrational forces at play in such cases. Not only are parents emotionally involved in these decisions but judges, lawyers, social workers, and guardians are also affected. While a child whose health is at risk represents our hope for the future, adults with disabilities, the mentally retarded adult whose health is also at risk, and the comatose nursing home patient represent our fears for the future. In dealing with our hopes—a healthy life—and our fears—a painful death without the ability to communicate with others—we are beginning to deal with the fabric of our social life in a technologically and scientifically sophisticated world.

Committing a Child to a Mental Hospital

The decision to commit a child to a mental hospital provides the foundation upon which to build an analytical framework. First and foremost, it involves a medical decision whose technological dimensions do not overwhelm us with claims to restore health. Neither does it destroy our understanding of what it means to be human. The decision to commit a child to a mental hospital appears, at least on the surface, less complicated morally and thus amenable to somewhat clearer legal guidance.

Less obvious but equally important is the recognition of the limits of human capacity brought by the decision to commit a child to a mental hospital. The circumstances in the child's life leading to this decision are usually tragic. We recognize all too quickly how painful they are to the child and his or her adult caretakers, but we often fail to acknowledge that the child's pain and our perception of that pain frequently cloud our vision and color our judgment. As a judge said in a landmark case involving legal procedures to be used when a child is committed, "In an earlier day, the problems inherent in coping with children afflicted with mental or emotional abnormalities were dealt with largely within the family."[1] This statement reflects the popular conception of the function of the family as an institution, one that is responsible for nurturing the physical and emotional well-being of its members.

At present, the decision to commit a child to a mental hospital takes place in a legal environment that sees "children's issues" and "medical issues" in a particular way, with contemporary perspectives on medical issues focusing on the rights of the patient as an individual rather than on the social and institutional setting of these issues. Similarly, there has been a growing tendency among some legal advocates to see the child, particularly the adolescent child, as an individual with rights separate from the family institution. Given these attitudes about law, medicine, and the family, it is not surprising that courts have had to struggle to determine proper legal response to requests for intervention and guidance.

Children are usually committed to state mental hospitals under provisions of the statutory schemes termed "voluntary" when the parent or guardian requests the commitment.[2] Litigation about the appropriateness of this type of commitment culminated in the *Parham* decision handed down by the U.S. Supreme Court in 1979. That lawsuit, brought on behalf of all the minors committed to the state mental hospitals in Georgia, was based on the theory that there must be some type of formalized legal procedure to review the parental decision to commit—and the hospital decision to accept—the child for hospital-based care. Since the statutory provision seemed to allow the hospital administrator to receive a minor for observation and diagnosis of mental illness if the parent or guardian requested it, the lawyers bringing the suit contended that the diagnostic stage of the process was tantamount to a finding of mental illness for purposes of commitment. Lawyers for the children argued that some type of hearing before an "impartial tribunal" should be required before the child could be committed. This legal theory was explicitly based on a landmark Court decision, *In re Gault,* which required an adversary hearing before a child could be committed to a juvenile institution.[3] This decision has served as the basis for any legal theory arguing for a child's legal rights, since the Court explicitly rejected the idea that the good-faith intentions of state officials involved in juvenile adjudication and disposition could replace the usual requirements of procedures derived from the constitutional guarantee of due process.[4]

Moreover, this legal theory was implicitly based on a mistrust of two institutions, medicine and the family. In the first instance, the suit suggested that the mental hospital could not be trusted to perform its social function without direct supervision by law. The children's lawyers believed that the hearing might create more political and social pressure to establish nonhospital-based places of treatment for mentally ill children. In the second instance, the theory implied that the family had not made its best effort to resolve the problems with the child before resorting to commitment to a mental hospital. One expert witness testified that some parents use mental hospitals as a dumping ground for their children but did not provide any direct evidence.[5] This lawsuit represents the prevailing view that there is an objective and rational decision that law ought to impose in this health care situation.

This assertion can be demonstrated by reviewing the facts of the commitment of one of the children involved in the suit. At the age of six, this child (referred to as J.L.) was admitted to a state mental hospital for an indefinite period at the request of his mother. Before admission, he had received outpatient hospital treatment. On the basis of information given at the time of admission, the admitting physician diagnosed the child as having a "hyperkinetic reaction to childhood." J.L.'s mother and his stepfather agreed to participate in family therapy while he was hospitalized, which meant that J.L. was permitted to go home for short visits. After two years of hospitalization, the child, then eight years old, was sent home to live with the parents but continued to attend school at the hospital. Within two months, the parents requested that J.L. be readmitted to the hospital, citing their inability to control him. Two years later the parents renounced their legal interests in the child, and he became a ward of the state. Several members of the hospital staff recommended that J.L. be placed in a special foster home with "a warm, supportive, and truly involved couple," but the social service agencies were unable to find such a placement; J.L. remained in the hospital.

One could assume that J.L.'s parents had made every effort and given up only after much soul-searching about his fate and that of the other members of the family. One might also contend, as did the lawyers bringing the lawsuit, that an impartial fact-finder might have come up with a different solution than that requested by the parents. This independent and objective solution would not be tainted by any ambivalence that the parents' decision might involve and could be imposed upon the parents even though, in their best judgment, the child's mental health would best be improved by hospitalization.

Chief Justice Burger, writing for the majority of the Court, rejected the theory proposed by the lawyers bringing the suit on behalf of the children in mental hospitals. While admitting that there was some risk of error in the parental decision to commit the child, the Court held that the review of the decision to admit should come after the admission to the hospital rather than before. By so doing, the Court legitimated many of the hospital-developed modes of control over parental and professional decision-making. Apparently, without any explicit directive from law, the hospitals had already developed a mental health care delivery network that included community clinics and specialized foster care homes. The difficulty that led to the lawsuit and created a moral dilemma was twofold: first, there simply were not enough of these facilities; second, those facilities that did exist were far from ideal in their capacity to heal. Can law adopt a certain posture, vis-à-vis resources and institutions outside of law, to facilitate meeting the needs of distressed children? The lawyers bringing the lawsuit believed that active legal intervention into parental and hospital decision-making would increase the sense of justice.

The Supreme Court's analysis forces us to deal with a host of issues that do not have clear rational solutions. On one level, the decision to commit a child to a mental hospital is, like other stereotypical parental decisions, "for the child's own good"; a parent, for instance, might decide that an adolescent daughter needs to live with her grandmother because she "gets into too much trouble" at home. Legal intervention, generally, would not be thought appropriate in such a decision. Consequently, there is no reason why placing the child in a mental hospital should change our attitude about the role of law, unless we thought the parents, in general, were unable to understand the course of treatment provided by the mental hospital's staff.

In the case of a parental decision to commit a child to a mental hospital, law should allow the parents to call upon institutionalized medicine to maintain the "health" of their child. The social-control function of medicine is performed by reviewing decisions after the fact. This is the appropriate form of legal supervision concerning the child's mental and emotional health, since parents are the primary caretakers. Even with the most sophisticated form of medical intervention we can imagine, society must rely on parents to provide the primary sustenance necessary for their children's mental and emotional health. Thus, one function of law in health care decisions for children is to recognize that there must be no objective or "right" answers in medical decisions.

Cancer Treatment for Minors

In recent years, a number of parents have sought alternative methods to conventional medicine when their children are faced with life-threatening illnesses.[6] One of the most celebrated of these cases in recent years is that of Chad Green,[7] who was under two years of age at the time he was diagnosed as having a form of childhood leukemia. Hospitalized, he began to receive the conventional treatment: chemotherapy. The entire program of treatment anticipated the use of cranial radiation at a future date, to which his parents had an aversion. After Chad spent a month in a midwestern hospital, his parents decided to move to Massachusetts, the father's home state. They took the child to a specialist at the world-renowned Massachusetts General Hospital who believed that cranial radiation would not be necessary. The parents told the physician that, in addition to the program of chemotherapy, they were themselves administering their own form of treatment, which consisted of distilled water, vegetarian foods, and high dosages of vitamins.

For the first several months during the intensive phase of the treatment, the parents were cooperative in carrying out the physician's instructions. They brought Chad to the hospital for his injections and apparently gave him the prescribed medication. As the treatment program entered the long-term maintenance phase, the parents, without telling the treating physician, stopped administering the medication. They apparently relied on their own treatment for more than three months before the physician discovered that they were no longer cooperating. After repeated efforts to persuade the parents to resume Chad's treatment, the physician convinced the hospital to bring a lawsuit to remove the decision-making authority from the parents. The highest court in Massachusetts ruled that the parents could not deny the child the necessary treatment. Since the lower court had ruled that they could retain physical custody as long as they obeyed the court's order, the parents took advantage of the limited jurisdiction of the courts of Massachusetts and left the state. The Greens eventually took Chad to Mexico, where the type of nutritional and metabolic treatment in which they believed is freely practiced. Chad Green died of leukemia nearly two years later.

Before we condemn the Greens as irresponsible parents, we ought to review some the "facts" about cancer treatment that makes their actions more understandable. As noted in chapter 3, chemical and radiation treatments are always a matter of percentages. We speak of a "cure" for cancer in a different manner, since remission—the present lack of any traceable sign of the disease—is the benchmark of success. Even among well-respected conventional practitioners there are differences of opinion about the extent of chemotherapy and radiation treatment that ought to be given in every case.

There are two possible ways of analyzing the legal implications of the parents' attitudes. First, the presumption of their right to make health care decisions for their children places an enormous burden on those who would like to override those decisions. Professor Joseph Goldstein (the co-author with Anna Freud and Albert Solnit of several books on law as it relates to children) stated this position most eloquently when he wrote:

> State supervention of parental judgment would be justified to provide any proven, non-experimental, medical procedure when its denial would mean *death* for a child who would otherwise have an opportunity for either a *life worth living* or a *life of relatively normal healthy growth* toward adulthood.[8]

Goldstein defends his position by arguing that, in any situation not met by his criteria for legal intervention, the parents should have the right to decide an issue that is inherently subjective regarding the child's health.

To apply Goldstein's criteria to such cases as Chad Green's seems to lead to morally ambiguous results. The difficulty arises because of the manner in which Goldstein interprets "nonexperimental." For Goldstein, the "medical profession" must agree that the proposed treatment is nonexperimental. In Chad Green's case, the proposed chemotherapy was not experimental, according to one of his oncologists.[9] The parents, however, did not have the same kind of scientific perspective on the problem of weighing the possible benefits against the probable risks that a medical professional has. On the one hand, they seemed to believe in the potential powers of medicine, but, on the other, they had an aversion to some of its techniques.

At one level, Goldstein's analysis is straightforward. There is no apparent scientific basis for the parents' beliefs, so it would be appropriate for law to intervene in order to give Chad a chance to mature until the time when law would allow him to make his own decisions. On another level, the bulk of Goldstein's work on health care decisions for children emphasizes family autonomy and indicates an uneasiness with a position that reinforces the values underlying prevailing medical practice.

If we accept the argument that cancer treatment for children is a special case and should thus be deemed "experimental," we would not applaud the result in the Chad Green case but rather condemn it as an unjustified intrusion upon parental decision-making authority. Under this view, radiation treatment and chemotherapy for a child would be considered experimental even though they are well established treatment protocols for leukemia in adults. Yet it is difficult to accept the almost-certain death of a child simply because we believe that law should respect parental autonomy. Thus, Goldstein's analysis seems to lead to moral ambiguity in its failure to confront explicitly the problems engendered by our highly sophisticated form of medicine.

What is wrong with Goldstein's approach is that he divides the objective from the subjective factors in health care decision-making for children, allocating authority for subjective considerations to the parents and the supposedly objective ones to medicine and law. Within the context of legal intervention, there can be no clear demarcation between the subjective and the objective factors involved in a controversy over a child's appropriate health care. In addition, Goldstein assumes that the child's life or death is somehow a separate phenomenon from his health.

The court's analysis fails to appreciate that the illness of a child is psychologically disorienting for families. As Robert Burt has pointed out in *Taking Care of Strangers,* a failure to take account of the social and psychological effects of a life-threatening illness may encourage law to become a brutalizing force in the face of moral and medical complexities. In its search for "objectivity" or "subjectivity," law could encourage individuals to inflict death on children.[10]

Kidney Transplantation Between Identical Twins

In this case, transplantation between identical twins, no one objected to the proposed donation by the healthy twin to the twin afflicted with an otherwise incurable kidney disease. No disagreements between the parents and the surgeons about the appropriateness of the risks involved for both children were alleged. All parties were in agreement about the apparent correctness of the decision from the medical point of view—a transplant between identical twins was preferable to that of a parent-to-child transplant. With so much apparent agreement, what conflict would form the basis of the lawsuit that ensued?[11]

The lawsuit was not based on any fundamental conflict of values concerning the health of either child but, rather, was aimed at reducing alleged legal uncertainty. Although the parents and the twins technically brought the lawsuit, the defendants—the physicians and the hospital—actually generated it by asserting their unwillingness to perform the operation without a court determination that the parents had the legal right to consent to the operation on behalf of both children. The lawsuit was thus a declaratory judgment action, one increasingly used in medical matters.

The lawsuit is all the more curious because there was very little doubt that the parents had the legal authority to consent to the transplantation on behalf of both children. What was perhaps doubtful was the moral correctness of the parents' decision and thus, by implication, the entire kidney transplantation program.

Kidney transplantation as a treatment makes certain assumptions about the social order. It assumes that some person either living or dead (by the new definition of brain dead) will provide a kidney for the ailing person as a gift. When medicine developed such a solution to an individual's kidney disease, there was very little discussion of the underlying moral compulsion that would be created when the prospective donor was "asked" for a kidney. Not only does the institution of modern medicine suggest the donor should "freely" give up a kidney, it also encourages families to pressure prospective donors within the family.[12]

Why does the assumption break down when the donor and recipient are children and identical twins, when from a medical point of view this type of transplant has the best chance of success? One portion of the answer lies in modern medicine's involvement in some degree of social as well as medical experimentation in developing the kidney transplantation program. In this case, medicine would be seeking legal validation of a social experiment.[13] Kidney transplantation is a *social* experiment in this particular case because transplants between identical twins involve little medical experimentation. In contrast, nonidentical twin kidney transplants still have a degree of medical "experimentation," since the problem of organ rejection has not been wholly resolved. But even in the usual cases of kidney transplantation, we do not yet know the full social implications, as, for example, the effect upon an adult sibling who provides a kidney that is rejected by the recipient after a few months.

The court could have made the moral ambiguity of the situation more visible for public discussion if it had simply declined to adjudicate and perhaps advised the parents to seek treatment by other physicians at a different hospital, if the present attending physicians and hospital continued to insist upon legal adjudication. The court could have pointed out that the moral correctness of the decision was a matter for resolution by the parents and any physicians engaged in transplantation.

Instead, the court suggested that the parents "would be able to substitute their consent for that of their minor children after a close, independent, and objective investigation of their motivation and reasoning."[14] Thus, the court insisted that its supervision was necessary without realizing that this assertion implied that the parents could not make the decision themselves. In fact, the court's proposed supervision became simply a matter of ensuring that the physicians followed all appropriate medical procedures before the operation. The court mentioned several times, for instance, that the physicians should establish through appropriate tests whether the twins were truly identical. The desire to supervise the entire process was derived from the court's need to justify its role when, in fact, there was no role for the court because there was no real conflict about the medical procedures proposed.[15]

Preserving the Health of Minors

Many cases involving the health of minors do not involve experimental procedures or treatment but present a host of ethical problems because of the underlying moral and emotional issues they raise.

Abortion for a Minor

Abortion for minors has generated a number of lawsuits challenging the constitutionality of various legislative enactments passed after the U.S. Supreme Court decision in 1973 legalizing abortions.[16] I shall not recount here the many court decisions dealing with the authority of legislatures to supervise health care decisions concerning the sexual behavior of children. Suffice it to say that the Supreme

Court of the United States has held as a matter of constitutional law that state legislatures cannot enact a statute that gives to parents, judges, or any third party the absolute right to veto the decision of a minor and her physician to abort a pregnancy.[17] Nor can the states enact statutes denying an abortion to a person under a certain age. The theoretical basis for the Court's idea of the right to an abortion is in large part dependent on biological functioning. Thus, if a person is biologically able to become pregnant, she has some legal right to have an abortion.

The challenge presented by the problem of abortion for minors is to develop a legal posture that recognizes both the biological and the social aspects of being a child or an adolescent in the latter part of the twentieth century. The Supreme Court's pronouncement on this problem achieved such a posture when it held constitutional a statute that required a physician to notify the parents of a minor before performing an abortion.[18] The opponents of the statute argued unsuccessfully that the statute was tantamount to giving the parents the power to veto the abortion and sought to enshrine the minor-physician relationship within a constitutional "right of privacy" doctrine developed by the Court.

The Court correctly upheld the statute because it believed that the parents could provide additional information about the psychological and medical background that would help the physician in exercising his medical discretion. The Court's finding is an example of sound policy-making for another reason. There is a need to exercise some control over physicians in what the Court describes as a "medical decision." Nevertheless, this is a curious description of the decision to terminate a pregnancy, since it confuses the procedure of termination with the process of decision-making.

We could assume that the moral problems we now associate with the termination of a pregnancy are somehow new problems, but for many years prior to the Court's decision there was plenty of evidence that women were obtaining abortions. These abortions were performed both by nonmedically trained persons and by physicians willing to risk criminal convictions.[19] In addition, by the time of the *Roe* v. *Wade*[20] decision, the elimination of criminal penalties for most abortions and the widespread use of contraceptive methods in the United States gave a clear indication that both men and women were concerned with the prevention of pregnancy. In this regard, medicine has been responsive and continues to engage in research into safer and more effective methods of contraception. Both prevention of conception and termination of the fetus's growth are apparently considered legitimate under a certain ill-defined but well-imagined set of circumstances. Given a lack of documentation concerning conception and abortion before 1973, it is easy for both supporters and opponents of the Court's decision in *Roe* to cite possible moral threats to the social fabric.

Nowhere is the tendency to use an imagined set of circumstances more pronounced than in the area of abortion for minors. Opponents of the Court's decision tend to draw a cinematic vision of a child who had perhaps engaged in sexual activity for the first time, is confused by her pregnancy, and is offered an abortion without any emotional and psychological support at a clinic supported by individuals who feel abortion is morally right. Supporters of the Court's decision present a picture of a young child who is pregnant and, without the emotional support of her parents, seeks out the abortion clinic. In this version of the story, the child fears severe emotional harm, if not physical harm, to herself if she tells her parents about the pregnancy and the planned abortion. The emotional intensity of both versions comes from the realization that someone heretofore considered a child has engaged in sexual activity and conception has occurred.

In the face of such emotional intensity, law ought to consider decisions in light of what is known rather than what is imagined. We know that medically trained persons are capable of performing abortions in a relatively safe manner and that a certain number of physicians are willing to perform these abortions. What is further known is that modern medicine is likely to be influenced by the research and development of techniques dealing with human reproduction. What was called a first-trimester abortion in 1973 will probably carry different moral and social implications in 1993.

Within that context, it becomes important to have some means of continually engaging the medical profession with the evolving social attitudes about fetal life. The parental notification requirement on the physician is one means of achieving that type of engagement. We can, of course, postulate that notifying the parents will, in many instances, create greater conflict for the minor and for the physician. But this conflict would provide a positive social function in that the physician would or would not proceed with the abortion in light of the social circumstances of the minor. Law cannot be used as a means of allowing physicians to treat abortion as a technical decision or, in their own terms, a "medical decision." A posture of law that required no contact with the parents would, in effect, allow the medical profession complete control over abortion procedures for minors.

A perspective that would validate a parental notification statute has the additional advantage of clarifying the moral issues involved in such cases where the wishes of the minor and the parents are at odds. Once it has been established that the parents have no absolute veto power over the minor's decision, the legal position is straightforward: a physician must obtain the "consent" of the minor. But the moral issues remain cloudy, because the conflict between the parent and the minor must be resolved in the physician's own mind before proceeding, unless he or she simply refuses to serve families in conflict over abortion. The physician is not entitled to turn to a judge for a resolution of the dilemma, since the legal "rights" are well defined, unless the parent claims that the child is incompetent and needs to have a guardian appointed to make the decision for her. The physician who chooses not to abort the pregnancy must conclude that he or she has no professional responsibility to provide services to a minor who may be unable or unwilling to nurture or care for a child. The physician who proceeds must enter into discussions with the parent and possibly face lawsuits.

The physician's preferred choice would be to engage the family in a conversation until a consensus can be reached. The child's reasons for wanting to move from conception to abortion must be weighed against other familial considerations. Within that milieu the physician must work toward a resolution.

The development of abortion clinics represents an important organizational advance for dealing with the full moral, political, and social ramifications of teenage abortions. Clinics are more likely than individual physicians to have available the counseling services for the teenager and her family that are often necessary before and after an abortion. In addition, the abortion clinic becomes the organizational basis for mobilizing the political and financial resources to provide abortion services to those without the necessary means to pay. And finally, at a time when there is so much conflict about abortion, the specialized clinic can become the organizational center for public debate about the related issues of adolescent sexuality, contraception, marriage, single parenthood, and abortion.

Heart Surgery for a Mentally Retarded Child

In a highly technological society, the health of a child with Down's syndrome is as emotional an issue as that of allowing a minor to have an abortion. The Down's syndrome case raises all our hopes and fears about our own cognitive ability in a society where rational behavior is so highly regarded. Furthermore, defining the meaning of health in regard to the Down's syndrome child is likely to become a matter of public debate because, until very recently, so many of these children spent a large portion of their lives in institutions.

A number of years ago a state court had to decide whether a twelve-year-old boy with Down's syndrome, who had been a resident of a state institution for the mentally retarded, should be given an operation to repair a defect in his heart. The proposed surgery was not necessary to save his life but was premised on the idea that the boy would become increasingly disabled by shortness of breath. The medical prognosis was that the child might live another twenty years without the operation. His parents refused to consent to the surgery, leading state welfare officials to initiate a lawsuit to have the boy declared neglected.[21]

The court had before it a child who, in one view of the facts, had apparently been abandoned by his parents to the state institution for care. In another view, the court heard evidence indicating that the proposed heart surgery was risky; the mortality rate was 5 to 10 percent, with more risk for a child with Down's syndrome because of postoperative complications. The court was correct in refusing to order the operation. The reasons can be more easily seen if we consider the institutional context of the decision.

The important factor for the court's consideration was the available realistic options, rather than some abstract notion of the "parents' rights" or the "best interests of the child." In this particular case, care of the child at risk was shared between a state institution for the mentally retarded and the parents. Even though the parents did not participate in daily care of the child, they had not abandoned him in any legal sense since they had not given up their legal rights and responsibilities.[22] Thus, they were entitled to be heard in determinations concerning the boy's health. Although the parents first had refused a diagnostic test—a catheterization—they later consented to it in order to determine the degree of damage to the child's pulmonary vessels. After the parents were given the medical diagnosis, they refused to consent to the proposed operation.

The state officials with daily responsibility for the child's care were also entitled to be heard, but their view still should not be controlling for two reasons. First, the operation is in itself dangerous. There was no clear indication that the risks were worth taking, although many parents would take such risks with children who do not have Down's syndrome. Second, and more important, the operation represents a potential break in the child's relationship with those outside the institution, his parents. The parents remain prepared to have a stake in the child's future, even from a distance. An operation against their will may break the fragile bond between them and their child.

Thus a situation arises in which the court is asked to choose between two definitions of health, one, perhaps pseudo-objective, in which the child's future is forecast in terms of statistical chances and probabilities, the other more qualitative and subjective. The court should side with the subjective view because it represents the kind of health we would want for ourselves and our own children. Otherwise, courts could perceive parents as interchangeable in the same ways that surgeons and physicians are interchangeable in terms of normative criteria. But a court must remember that the obligations parents feel toward their children are not the same as the social obligations of a health care professional. The surgeon who might perform the operation has no continuing relationship with the child, nor does a volunteer who works with the child daily replace the broad social obligation that the parents usually have.

Considerable media attention was directed at this particular case, but the parents never responded to media inquiries.[23] The subsequent refusal to allow the operation in the context of the medical facts is unreasonable only if we assume there is a single objective standard for judging which risks should be taken to protect the health of children.

Conclusion

In the last few years we have seen a growing number of legal pronouncements regarding the health care of children. Since courts, legislatures, and administrative agencies speak in terms of "rights," we may have incorrectly assumed that law can provide us with a moral directive of what should be done. The emphasis on "rights" has encouraged us to try to impose one view of health that has led to an increasing tendency to see health care decisions as objective.

What we really need, however, is a legal model of health care decision-making that allows for fundamental distinctions, distinctions that in turn would help us to understand and resolve the moral dilemmas presented by modern medicine. We must stop idealizing the manner in which health care for children is provided. Once the family decides it needs additional help in preserving the health of its child, it must move into a new organizational context that includes the hospital, the institution for the mentally retarded, and the abortion clinic. The move from family-centered health care to institution-centered health care increases the potential for conflicting definitions of health. In most instances the parents' view of health will predominate. But in situations such as those involving abortion and contraception, some parents will have to face deep conflicts with their own values, their concepts of their children, and their ideas of the future. Law has begun to recognize that the ability to procreate, in and of itself, allows a minor to decide on her own whether to terminate pregnancy through abortion.

The second distinction that a legal model of health care decision-making would require is a definition of the social obligations of health care professionals toward incompetents. At some point, in looking at health rather than treatment, we must acknowledge that professional obligations have limits and thus professional authority to decide must have limits as well.

We live in a world in which different views about health are becoming increasingly more visible. By looking at these conflicting views of health through the perspective of modern scientific medicine, we see health and the potential for healing in only one light— the intervention of modern medicine. But healing involves a much larger conception since it also denotes something beyond the physical, a holistic sense of human life. As these conflicts develop, law will be asked to intervene more and more. Law can play a more useful role if it takes an institutional approach to issues such as the call in 1983 to regulate the health care decisions of children of Christian Scientists.[24] A legal system devoted to the concept of justice would never develop such an approach. We must move away from using neglect and abuse statutes in dealing with medical issues for children, since these mask the essential value conflicts. Such legislation must specifically deal with the issue of whether the treatment of children should be subjected to the same approach as the treatment of other incompetents.

What we need, then, is some type of mediating role for law, which would mean, in many instances, an unwillingness to respond to the call for its intervention. In Chad Green's case, for instance, the most desirable process would encourage the parents and the attending physician to consider carefully not only the health care needs of the child at risk but also their own attitudes toward illness, death, and the dark side of their individual futures. For such a process to be possible, a radical change would be required in our present approach to legal intervention in conflicts between care providers and physicians over health care for incompetents.

First, there needs to be special legislation that addresses health care decisions for children. We have too often used the rubric of parental neglect, with its attendant moral overtones, to justify legal intervention in medical decisions. The use of the child neglect and abuse statute has meant that all lawsuits start by assuming the parents are "bad," an assumption not warranted in such cases as that of Chad Green's. Such proposed legislation must take into account the prevailing ethos of modern scientific medicine. It should contain the following three elements: (1) an assumption in favor of parental decision-making, (2) a presumption against legal intervention, and (3) a process for determining the nature of the controversy.

The first requirement is designed to encourage physicians and judges to listen carefully to parents before authorizing a certain type of action based on a medical-legal sense of professional duty. The second requirement is important because the assumption has developed that medical decisions are entitled to preview, whereas most other important moral decisions are not. The third requirement is necessary because many parents who object to conventional treatment for their offspring often have alternative views toward the nature of healing.

This proposed legislation would enhance the role of the court as mediator by suggesting in the majority of cases that there is no legal controversy, although there may be a great moral controversy that requires dialogue about the nature of caring. Such dialogue should be encouraged by law because it in fact calls upon us for the greatest of human effort.

Chapter 7

The Path Toward Caring and Justice

Under existing legal analysis, the greatest impediment to modernizing our notion of caring and justice is the very existence of the malpractice system. The prospect of patients suing their physicians for the failure to undertake a certain diagnosis or explain remote risks of a medical procedure, particularly surgery, has resulted in the practice of defensive medicine and a general deterioration in the idealized view of the doctor-patient relationship. Jury awards of large sums in damages in highly publicized medical malpractice suits appear to many to be perverse, if not unjust. Judges have suggested that the possibility of a malpractice suit could lead physicians to make "wrong" decisions in cases of critically ill patients. These same judges have thus constructed a form of immunity from malpractice liability to advance the physician's healing function.

The legal malpractice system needs to be subjected to close scrutiny because it is the starting point of current legal analysis of medicine. Then, if it turns out that our modern problems with medicine are not alleviated by major or minor reform of the malpractice system, it will be apparent that other aspects of legal and medical institutions are in need of reform. Under an institutional approach, we also need to examine related issues such as the way we deal with death within the legal system, changes in the education of both physicians and lawyers, and the moral and political implications of financing health care in the United States.

Malpractice Reform

Any discussion of malpractice reform must confront the overriding sense that something is awry in our use of law. We think of litigation involving medical matters either as wrong, since it represents an unnecessary and costly battle between patients and physicians, or inadequate as a means of supervising unethical or incompetent doctors. However, we must treat these misperceptions as indications of the need to rethink the relationship of law and medicine. If, for instance, we compare the role of liability rules in medicine and automobile accidents, we would find little to support the claim that new innovations in American medical malpractice law are too favorable to the victims of medical accidents.[1]

Foremost in the examination of complaints about the medical malpractice system is the claim that malpractice leads to the defensive practice of medicine. This complaint indicates that many individuals, including physicians, have begun to treat law as the source of professional ethics rather than as a guide to professional duty. Too often the proposed legal reforms are designed merely to allow physicians to maintain their philanthropic view of themselves rather than seek a new vision of the modern healer.

Physicians who call for a system that would prevent patients from suing them in all but the most blatant instances of negligent care have assumed that a philanthropic vision of their professional roles is sufficient to answer all ethical questions. They disregard the transformations of individual conceptions of health, life, and death that occur in response to cultural changes. Physicians have yet to realize that these changes, caused in part by progress in biomedical research, will require them to make radical alterations in their understanding of the roles they perform in society. With the advent of new drugs, complex diagnostic techniques, and more sophisticated modes of intervention, patients have shifted their faith from the physician to technological tools. The malpractice suit, then, is the symptom, rather than the cause, of the problem of the lack of congruence between physicians' conceptions of their social role and the changing expectations of society.

A recent set of proposed legislative reforms, designed to check the rise of physician malpractice premiums in New York State, illustrates how the current legal debate centers on symptoms rather than causes. During the negotiations between the New York Medical Society (representing the physicians), the governor, and legislative leaders, physicians insisted that the legislature limit the amount of damages that patients could recover for "pain and suffering." This proposed legislation was seen as a means of reducing potential damage awards and thus slowing the rise in malpractice insurance premiums. In proposing the limitation, the physicians were apparently viewing illness and its consequences from what they considered a scientific perspective. They thought it was perfectly reasonable to propose that an objective amount of pain and suffering resulting from any medical misadventure could be determined in advance and thus fixed by the legislature. From their perspective, the jury's authority to assess the amount of pain and suffering in each case appeared irrational and unjust.

In rejecting this particular request, the governor argued that the proposed limitation would be unfair to the victims of medical accidents as compared to victims of other kinds of accidents which carry no such limitations. For example, the amount of money for pain and suffering that a victim of an automobile accident can receive is set by juries in individual cases rather than by the legislature. Significantly enough, the physicians apparently did not realize that their proposed reform, if adopted, implied a wholesale reform of the American legal system of litigation about accidents.[2]

The simplest and most popular explanation of large jury awards is that society has become antagonistic toward physicians; we no longer trust them, and we welcome the opportunity to punish them with arbitrary awards for pain and suffering. This explanation readily leaps to mind if we see the interaction of law and medicine as a battle. Large awards that might be thought inconsistent with existing standards, however, have been reduced either by judges or by agreement between the parties after the award. In fact, if the size of the award is clearly inconsistent with existing legal standards, the physician's lawyer has every incentive to ask the trial judge to set aside the award and to appeal to higher courts if his request is denied. Agreement is the more likely choice, because a lawyer would prefer to negotiate the amount downward than to have a judge reduce it.[3]

The more likely explanation for what physicians describe as "too large awards" in malpractice suits has to do with modern medical misadventure. While there have been tremendous gains in treating disease as a result of the more intrusive forms of medical intervention, the adverse cases, be they inherent risks of the procedures or results of professional negligence, are often seen as tragic.

There are several reasons for this response. First, as the success rate for a given medical procedure rises, the failed cases appear especially tragic and thus painful. When a much greater percentage of women died in childbirth and fewer at-risk babies survived, it was easier to view medical misadventure or a less-than-perfect result as one of life's inherent risks. A second consequence of medical success is that patients who might have died fifty years ago survive today. A small percentage of these survivors live with severe impairments that juries may consider to be the responsibility of medicine.

Another aspect of the problem is medical specialization and the concurrent growth in medical knowledge. As more and more is known about the prevention of medical misadventure during childbirth, for instance, our attitudes toward less-than-perfect results change. Forty years ago it was common practice in hospital deliveries to sedate patients heavily. Although that procedure was in accordance with prevailing medical practice, it is now known to create risks to the baby and mother. In addition, as obstetrics has grown as a specialty, what is expected of the physician assisting in childbirth has also grown. The knowledge of the general practitioner, who delivered many babies a mere forty years ago, is no longer sufficient by modern medical standards.

This growth in knowledge is a two-edged sword. On the one hand, a large number of at-risk babies survive and more difficult pregnancies end in successful childbirth. On the other hand, some of those at-risk babies and difficult pregnancies are not totally successful, and the damages appear great to physicians, families, and lawyers. Another consequence of this enormous growth in knowledge is that some physicians are simply unable to keep pace with the rapid changes in their fields and thus may not be able to screen out those cases that are beyond their competence.

The cumulative effect of these large jury awards for malpractice may be to change the actual delivery of health care services. There are some indications that physicians are starting to leave the specialty of obstetrics.[4] It might be true that malpractice insurance costs and malpractice litigation are leading them to other specialties. But we should consider whether other factors might not also be encouraging a shift away from this specialty. One factor possibly affecting obstetricians' degree of job satisfaction is the increasing trend of active patient and father/familial participation in childbirth. This means that in the normal course of events, in which there is no medical misadventure or complications, the obstetrician no longer deals solely with the patient. The physician is constantly drawn into the social context of the patient's life through the familial participation in office visits and labor and actual delivery. Physicians uncomfortable with sharing knowledge with patients or with the presence of another person who observes their manners and techniques may simply be uncomfortable with the doctor's changing professional role. Now that the mystery surrounding the medical role in childbirth has been dispelled, some professionals may be ill at ease with their less authoritative position.

At the heart of the medical malpractice issue is the relationship of liability to insurance. The effect of imposing liability where there is insurance is to socialize the cost of the accident, since all patients eventually pay higher fees. As a result, the awarding of pain and suffering damages in malpractice cases is a way of including the social costs of an individual patient's pain and suffering in the total cost of the medical enterprise.

One reform that could make the medical malpractice system more equitable would be to introduce the possibility of organizational, rather than individual, professional liability. Claims against physicians could be transformed into claims against the hospital for failure to supervise physicians properly. This is particularly true when physicians are using intrusive and innovative treatments, such as artificial heart transplants, that are experimental. In such a legal change, the hospital would be viewed as more representative of the social institution of medicine than is the individual physician. In a recent reform, for example, the New York legislature adopted such an approach by requiring hospitals to provide a certain amount of malpractice insurance coverage for physicians who practice in their facilities.[5] We may find that we have to experiment with various ways of dealing with the issue of liability before we find the best social solution.

Health Care Delivery and Legislative Reform

Once we free ourselves from the prevailing attitude concerning malpractice and accept the possibility of litigation as a social good, we can see the need for legislative reform in two other areas: death and health care decision-making for children.

Attitudes Toward Death

To confront the issue of death, I suggest, first, that legislatures resist the trend toward living wills. Instead, we should increase our conscious efforts to understand the changing social context of death. Legislatures should enact measures to encourage the building of hospices. These measures would include licensing provisions, guidelines for Medicare eligibility, and coverage of some form of hospice care through private insurance. Second, legislatures should enact statutes specifically authorizing hospital control over physicians' actions concerning critically ill patients. Finally, legislatures should enact statutes describing the circumstances under which physicians may be held criminally liable.

In all these legislative enactments, our way of thinking about these issues must be changed. Rather than the usual academic discourses on death and dying, we must reaffirm the social obligations of individuals to care for those who are critically ill and disabled. Although individuals live longer today than at any other time in our history, death is still inevitable. Our present preoccupation with dying is not socially healthy because it focuses on the termination of active social connections at a time when we should be increasing our capacity to care for the growing number of disabled and critically ill people. The progress in changing attitudes toward death will necessarily be slow in comparison to fifty years ago, since there is so much greater capacity to arrest infection, to resuscitate, and to intervene with more refined surgical techniques.

Unfortunately, with so much discussion of "natural" death and concern that physicians misuse their technology to prolong life needlessly, legislatures must be careful not to give in to romantic and antitechnological visions of caring. We have knowledge about biological function that cannot be reversed. The issue is our use of that knowledge in actual health care delivery. We also need to resist the tendency of scientists to believe religiously in the inevitability of progress—that a cure for cancer will surely be found, that artificial organs can be perfected and made available to all who need them, even that aging and death will be overcome.

Even more important than new legislation dealing with death is a reevaluation of the function of medicine itself. It is time we distinguished our social value for the preservation of human life from medical professionals' claims that they are the "preservers of life." Such transcendental claims on the part of physicians have encouraged judges to assume similar omniscient powers when they are called upon to decide who should live or die.

The Care of Children

This need for a reorientation of our perspective concerning the function of medicine can be best understood if we take as the ultimate test of medical-legal interaction the care of children, rather than that of the terminally or critically ill. Legal involvement in health care decisions for children, and by implication for other legal incompetents, raises fundamental questions about the evolving meanings of health and caring. While the family rather than medicine is the institution with primary responsibility for providing care for children in our society, the involvement of medicine presents a possible conflict about the meaning of care. This conflict arises because organizations—hospitals, clinics, cancer wards, and other caretaking facilities such as those for the mentally retarded—provide a form of institutionalized care. While its importance should not be underestimated, institutionalized care, unlike family care, does not provide the affective bonds that are the foundation of our social fabric.

Thus, in all the present clamoring for legislation, we cannot forget the need for legislation to establish a new model of health care decision-making for children. Using this model, courts would resist the temptation to play God and focus instead on their role as the protector of our sense of communal values. Courts would assume a mediating rather than adjudicative role, although they would still be the final arbiters, in line with their function as the ultimate repository of society's values.

There is a certain amount of inevitable indeterminacy in law when it encounters medicine and other basic social institutions such as the family. This indeterminacy in law in the face of the institution of the family is beneficial to the society. It helps to make clear the importance of those factors in the social fabric that bind individuals to each other. The Baby M case illustrates this point: Within the nexus of caring, justice, and the family, Baby M's custody could have been assigned either to her biological mother or to the sperm donor—the father—and his wife. The fact that the New Jersey Supreme Court awarded custody to the father and his wife and visitation rights to the biological mother is secondary to the grounds on which the court did so. The court rejected the trial judge's view of the case as one involving contractual entitlements and constitutional rights. Rather, the court, in a case involving modern biomedical technologies, emphasized that there are some kinds of agreements between apparently consenting adults that the law will not specifically enforce. By using legal doctrines associated with adoption, termination of parental rights, putative parents, and child custody, the court made visible for public debate and discussion many of the social and moral implications of institutionalized medicine's willingness to provide opportunities for "surrogate parenting."[6] We may have the medical expertise to foster surrogacy, but that knowledge alone does not mean that its application is in line with our present social views on reproduction. The Baby M case is a clear example of how the law can side with prevailing communal values and at the same time encourage debate on the possible moral consequences of rapidly advancing medical expertise.

Educational Reform

We are going to face some difficult choices concerning procedures for health care delivery. With an institutional approach, we might begin to think first and foremost about health rather than progress in medicine. "Health" implies not just the delivery of technical services but active social participation, which must include both physicians and potential patients. While many public choices will make a marginal impact in changing our present orientation toward medical issues—such as the adoption by judges and legislators of the perspective argued for throughout this book, cost containment measures, changes in federal support for health care, and even modification of malpractice insurance plans or programs—ultimately change must begin with the education of physicians, lawyers, and other professionals.

This change must first occur where all professional groups are educated together—in college and university undergraduate programs. A large percentage of college students enrolled in undergraduate programs at our leading universities are headed toward some type of professional or graduate program upon graduation.[7] Until recently the response of college educators to this phenomenon was to try to ensure that future professionals were exposed to such traditional humanities subjects as philosophy, literature, and history. Today's college students live in a technologically sophisticated world, where specialization and expertise are highly prized even within the university. The undergraduate, whose professional orientation may have been formed as early as his or her entrance to college, often treats humanities and social science requirements as obstacles to be overcome and thus irrelevant to the true purpose of education.

What is needed at the undergraduate level is a frank acknowledgment that today's students see themselves as future professionals. The meaning of "professional" is unclear, as the word today has connotations ranging from the historical religious one of someone who "professes his or her religious belief" to someone with a narrow and highly specialized view of issues—a meaning that is at its base anti-intellectual. As such, from a very early stage today's undergraduates have a special relationship to knowledge and expertise vis-à-vis others in society. The university and college must begin to educate undergraduates to see reality from a variety of perspectives; as future doctors, lawyers, engineers, scientists, and business men and women, these citizens are likely to face problems that involve the intersections of social, legal, scientific, and medical issues.

One way in which this new educational perspective could be introduced is for colleges and universities to develop interdisciplinary programs that would allow students to synthesize knowledge from various disciplines in solving problems. These would not simply be courses in which faculty from different disciplines participate, nor would they be courses in applied ethics. Rather, they would be courses in which, before teaching the courses, the instructors would have consulted with colleagues from a variety of disciplines on the problems to be discussed in the courses. By engaging in such discourses, the instructors would broaden their frameworks for teaching students about important social problems. Students in their undergraduate years would learn that, in order for their knowledge or expertise to be socially useful, their approaches must include perspectives from a variety of disciplines. By teaching beyond his or her discipline, the university professor would be performing a form of public service by providing tomorrow's citizenry with an understanding of the limits of overly specialized approaches to modern problems.

The training and education of physicians must be refocused toward a notion of preserving health. In addition, emphasis might be placed on preventive medicine and other issues that are germane to maintaining the community's well-being. The institutional approach to medicine would make physicians more able to engage in a partnership with their patients in a joint search for health.

These proposed changes in medical education do not assume that a scientific orientation to disease would be lost. Instead, this education would increase the capacity of future medical professionals to understand the perspectives of others, including patients, regulators, and legal professionals, who increasingly interact with medicine as an institution.

The most dramatic effect of proposed changes in legal education would be to educate future lawyers and judges to make decisions in the face of uncertainty. The recent interaction of medicine and scientific theory has demonstrated that lawyers' preoccupation with facts has left them ill-equipped to deal with undetermined circumstances. Lawyers generally assume that increasing certainty on the part of law is necessarily more socially useful than is uncertainty. In general, legal training must allow future lawyers to understand that law is dependent on other social institutions and that professional education generally needs to be reexamined in light of the crisis in professionalism we are experiencing in our society.[8]

Interdisciplinary courses and clinical courses within law schools have traditionally sought to perform this function. Most of them, however, remain outside the core curriculum; they are thought of as "adding depth" rather than being an integral part of the training of lawyers. Furthermore, the model of clinical education in law school has been built on the false premise that medical education, supposedly because of its greater scientific basis, offers the appropriate model for clinical legal education. We must start to understand that being a professional is not simply an extension of scientific knowledge but part of artistry.[9]

Being a practicing professional is participating in both science and art. The artistic image is presented here because we are in need of a new image and definition of professionalism in this society that helps professionals think about the intrinsic worth of their tasks. Too much of our discussion of professionalism is concerned with the professional's autonomy and his or her contractual relationship to clients. The professional, much like the artist who creates a work of art, should see encounters with human beings as having intrinsic worth for both the professional and the client. Those human beings who are the recipients of the professional's many years of continuing self-learning through formal education and practice cannot be "pre-arranged." People do not have scripts for communicating about matters of life and death. Rather, the professional must hold himself or herself out as available to serve the individuals and the social issues facing the particular profession at any given moment in time. Professionals thus care for their clients as part of their own life's work.[10]

While they represent an important start, ideally these interdisciplinary perspectives on the problems law encounters would appear in the core curriculum. The case method of legal instruction can easily be used to illustrate these perspectives as well as to present professional students with opportunities to work with instructors in resolving the seemingly intractable problems that society faces.

Financing Health Care

The most profound discovery likely to emerge from legislative examination of ways to reform malpractice is the dysfunction created by the way we finance health care in the United States. Many of the largest claims of malpractice involve situations that in other Western countries are covered by national health insurance programs or other forms of social insurance. Our present method of financing health care delivery does not cover the social and economic costs of all cases, including cases of medical misadventure, regardless of whether anyone can be said to be legally at fault.

Lawyers, medical educators, and scholars from many disciplines must begin to examine carefully the kind of health care system we have in the United States. Such an examination should be comparative and multidisciplinary. Several scholars have argued that there ought to be a "right to health" as the first step to resolving issues such as the need for financing the care of those afflicted with a "catastrophic disease."[11] These studies are useful in the legislative debates because they help to emphasize that health should be thought of in social as opposed to scientific terms. But they are not definitive for law because they cannot resolve the jurisprudential issues of what "rights" mean in law.

One of these studies, by a philosopher, makes the compelling point that it is intuitively obvious that one has a duty to come to the aid of others as the basis for a right to health care. But the study fails to ask why law in America has never sanctioned the failure of people to do so.[12] We need a more thorough analysis of this question, beyond the "individualism" of the American character. Such an explanation would require us to understand that entitlement might be defined for law not in terms of social duties to others but of who will prevail in a conflicting situation.[13] Thus, the failure to award damages in general when someone fails to come to the aid of another may require judgments about when it is appropriate to compel the transfer of money through law. Despite the position of law as developed by judges, legislators could extend health care benefits in the form of insurance reimbursement to a host of individuals presently not covered by private or public programs. My point is a simple one. In the context of our legal system in which courts play the ultimate role in resolving individual disputes and interpreting the legality of statutes, legal scholars should avoid "rights" language in favor of an institutional perspective on issues related to health care.

As we study health care systems from a comparative perspective, it is apparent, for instance, that the method of financing health care in the United States has tremendous effects on the system of health care delivery. The traditional method of examining this problem has been to look at various financing programs or plans. A more useful method of study, one that is in line with an institutional approach, might be to study the effect of financing schemes when medicine is interacting with some other basic institution, such as law.

A recent decision in Great Britain rejecting the doctrine of informed consent in a malpractice suit illustrates the kind of comparative and interdisciplinary examination I recommend. In that case, *Sidaway* v. *Board of Governors of the Bethlem Royal Hospital and others,*[14] the House of Lords rejected what it called the "American" doctrine of informed consent, which would have required the physician, a neurosurgeon, to inform the plaintiff patient of the inherent or remote risks of paralysis as a result of an operation on her spine. Instead, the House of Lords adopted the precedent set in *Bolam,* an English case that upheld that "a doctor is not negligent if he acts in accordance with a practice accepted at the time as proper by a responsible body of medical opinion even though other doctors adopt a different practice."[15] Before concluding that the House of Lords' rejection indicates that the American doctrine of informed consent is unworkable, it is worth noting the distinctive social setting in which *Sidaway* occurred and how it differs from its American counterpart.

Mrs. Sidaway was a patient in a Western country with a national health service program. Examining the case from an interdisciplinary perspective, we might wonder if the particular kind of health care delivery system in the United Kingdom might not have led the

English judges to see the role of law in relation to medicine in a different light from our American judges.[16]

From an institutional perspective, we would not ask whether English and American law differ on the relevance of informed consent in malpractice litigation. Instead we would focus on the relationship of malpractice to health care delivery. From such a perspective we might expand our inquiry to include a comparison of health care delivery to malpractice litigation in countries with legal and health care systems different from our own. For instance, since France and the United States have different legal systems as well as different health care delivery systems, it might be useful to look at issues that would focus our attention on the interaction of these systems in each country. Law, like medicine, is part of a nation's social context. In addition, a study of how different legal systems respond to the problem of medical misadventure would lead students to think about broader issues, such as how different societies conceive of authority, how professionals operate under these varied conceptions, and how policymakers respond differently to similar problems in view of their national restraints.

Such a comparative perspective would shed new light on emerging health care issues such as cost containment at a time when a large proportion of our society is becoming older and more disabled and is using health care services more frequently. The Catastrophic Health Care bill enacted in 1988 that provides such protection for the elderly[17] is likely to help fuel the growing debate about health care costs and the inadequacies of our health care delivery system in providing care for other groups such as children and the unemployed. We might discover that we must find new definitions and receptacles of liability for medical misadventures. For example, Medicare's methods of containing costs through diagnostic related groups (the practice of assigning a fixed amount to any given procedure, regardless of how many tests a physician requests or the length of stay in the hospital) create incentives for hospitals that might appear contrary to the physicians' standards for quality care.[18] "Surrogate parenting" clearly involves law, medicine, and the family as institutions. It also involves individuals only imagined—technologists, medical and legal personnel, and extended family members. One can envision possible future scenarios that include litigation involving laboratory workers, psychologists, genetic counselors, legal advisers, and grandparents. The projected issues point, yet again, to the crucial nexus of law, medicine, and the family as institutions. There are public policy alternatives that legislatures or courts could devise that take account of the nexus and would allow for some form of surrogate parenting to develop without the likelihood of increased litigation.

Malpractice is the negative side of law seen in its larger social context. Seeing problems from the institutional viewpoint does not provide textbook answers to them, but the perspective does offer a starting point, a way of thinking about the problems that also considers the social and economic costs. Acquired Immune Deficiency Syndrome (AIDS) is a case in point. AIDS is so troubling because it is a chronic condition that tests our ability to care. Furthermore, as we reflect upon the way in which we have viewed the at-risk groups, and even the way we have classified the disease as "sexually transmitted,"[19] we are reminded of the need to think of health as a social construct as we face issues of how much to spend on research on AIDS as opposed to other diseases, whether physicians are entitled to breach confidentiality, whether patients can sue physicians in order to compel them to offer some form of treatment or amelioration, and how to pay for the care. While the perspective offered here provides no ready answer to the AIDS dilemma, it does help us open up for discussion the basic classification of the disease as "sexually transmitted" or as a "terminal disease." Such classifications involve stigmas of some kind and allow us to ignore the challenge of devising ways of caring for persons in chronic conditions. Furthermore, it makes us more cautious in the use of law as a response to the fears that AIDS creates. Given the uncertainty created by modern medicine, that alone is no small measure of success.

Notes

Introduction: The Search for Caring and Justice

1. See Shirley Lindenbaum, *Kuru Sorcery: Disease and Danger in the New Guinea Highlands* (Palo Alto, Calif.: Mayfield Publishing Co., 1979). We often lose sight of the rite of passage of death in our highly scientific society; for instance, we see ill health or the threat of death as requiring a response from others surrounding the sick or dying person. Incorporation of the ideas of modern biology into an individual's own belief systems and attitudes about illness and death is a matter of social or cultural transformation. Larry Churchill, in *Rationing Health Care in America* (Notre Dame, Ind.: University of Notre Dame Press, 1987), provides an excellent assessment of most of the modern liberal theories of justice as applied to medical ethics. His social conception of justice helps to inform the perspective of this book.

2. The importance of financial arrangements to institutionalized medicine is best illustrated by the fact that we often rely on financial incentives to control costs or achieve social health goals such as "prevention."

3. Robert A. Burt, *Taking Care of Strangers: The Rule of Law in Doctor-Patient Relations* (New York: Free Press, 1979), pp. 124–27. Burt argues that it is false to assume that decision-making can be properly vested in any single individual (doctor, patient, or judge) and that law must not intervene to give this exclusive power to individuals, thereby creating certainty where none in fact exists. Instead, law should create the framework for in-depth dialogue between the parties; it "should keep the parties off-balance, uncertain about the precise measure of their power or impotence regarding one another, in order to counterbalance the impulse toward destructively stereotypical choicemaking/choiceless role allocations that inevitably arise from the stressful confusions of their situation" (p. 140).

4. Jay Katz, *The Silent World of Doctor and Patient* (New York: Free Press, 1984), pp. 82–84.

5. Churchill comments (*Rationing,* p. 117) that the British National Health Service provides health care as a basic right of all citizens, thereby promoting an expectation of health care which differs from that in the United States. An innate sense of egalitarianism pervades the British system, which creates a greater understanding of medical misadventures on the part of the health care professional and the patients.

6. See William F. May, *The Physician's Covenant: Images of the Healer in Medical Ethics* (Philadelphia: Westminster Press, 1983), pp. 146–49.

7. The best evidence of this divergence are studies indicating that a large percentage of patients do not follow their doctor's prescriptions or orders as to how to care for their illness. While this failure to comply might be explained by the failure or inability of laypersons to understand the complexities of scientific language of modern medicine, the best explanation of this breakdown in communication lies in an analysis of the fundamental aspects of doctor-patient relationships under modern conditions. See Katz, *Silent World,* p. xiv; May, *Physician's Covenant,* pp. 151–52.

8. With a social and relational perspective, health is best thought of as a continuum rather than a delimited biological state. With the continuum notion of health, we also come to understand that a person with kidney disease, for instance, may need a level of care from health professionals and family members that is different from that needed by a person with the symptoms of a common cold. In the latter case, the level of care necessary to restore health may be as simple as bed rest and sympathy, assuming these symptoms do not mask a more life-threatening disease. In the former case, the level of care may involve a whole range of medical interventions (from dialysis to organ transplantation) and numerous professionals and laypersons.

Chapter 1: Liability Rules and the Entitlement to Health

1. Liability rules are legal provisions that allow one party who is injured by the conduct of another to force the injuring party to pay monetary damages.

2. See, e.g., Norman Daniels, *Just Health Care* (Cambridge: Cambridge University Press, 1985).

3. As we deal with law it is important to think in terms of conflicts—who will prevail in the event of a contest—rather than abstract notions of rights. Those writers who use the notion of rights admit readily that rights are limited and never absolute, but they fail to note the important question of when those so-called rights are limited by the society through the institution of law.

4. *In re Quinlan,* 70 N.J. 10, 49, 355 A. 2d 647, 668 (1976).

5. For instance, we do not yet require airbags in all automobiles, al-

though such devices would clearly save lives. See Guido Calabresi, *Ideals, Beliefs, Attitudes, and the Law* (Syracuse, N.Y.: Syracuse University Press, 1985), p. 89.

6. 42 U.S.C.A. § 273–274 (West Supp. 1988).

7. Guido Calabresi and A. Douglas Melamed, "Property Rules, Liability Rules, and Inalienability: One View of the Cathedral," *Harvard Law Review* 85, no. 6 (April 1972): 1111–15.

8. Calabresi, *Ideals*, p. 88.

9. I am indebted to Guido Calabresi's in-depth exploration of approaches to health care entitlements. See Guido Calabresi and Philip Bobbitt, *Tragic Choices* (New York: W. W. Norton & Co., 1978), pp. 186–91. Calabresi states that the costs of medical services such as transplants may heavily influence which medical options are pursued. See Guido Calabresi, "The Problem of Malpractice: Trying to Round Out the Circle—Parts I & II," *Toronto Law Journal* 27 (1977): 131–37.

10. The Admissions and Policies Committee of the Seattle Artificial Kidney Center (Seattle God Committee) determined appropriate recipients according to factors that included age, sex, marital status, dependents, income, net worth, psychological stability, past performance, and future potential. Seven representatives of different segments of society made up the committee, which met from 1961 until 1967. See Calabresi and Bobbitt, *Tragic Choices*, pp. 187–88.

11. 42 U.S.C. § 426(h) (1983).

12. See Uniform Anatomical Gift Act (U.L.A.) (West 1968). Organ procurement has been addressed with the adoption of the act in all fifty states.

13. See comments to the revised Uniform Anatomical Gift Act § 2 (1987) (West Supp. 1988). Subsection (h) makes explicit the intention of the original act, "that an individual has the right to dispose of his body without subsequent veto by others." The revised Section 2(h) states, "An anatomical gift that is not revoked by the donor before death is irrevocable and does not require the consent or concurrence of any person after the donor's death."

14. See Prefatory Note to Uniform Anatomical Gift Act (1987).

15. *Organ Transplantation,* Report of the Task Force on Organ Transplantation (Washington, D.C.: U.S. Department of Health and Human Services, April 1986).

16. Note that the law on organ donations required new definitions of death since by traditional cardiocirculatory definitions the accident victim is not dead. Unresponsiveness to external stimuli and internal need, an absence of spontaneous muscular movements or spontaneous respiration, and no elicitable reflexes indicate brain death; these criteria cover brain-stem activity as well as higher brain functions. See Alexander M. Capron

and Leon R. Kass, "A Statutory Definition of the Standards for Determining Human Death: An Appraisal and a Proposal," *University of Pennsylvania Law Review* 121, no.1 (November 1972): 89–90.

17. Uniform Anatomical Gift Act § 8(b) (1987).

18. Note that a person could not force someone to "give" human body parts even if needed to preserve his or her life. See, e.g., *Head* v. *Colloton*, 331 N.W. 2d 870 (Iowa 1983), leukemia victim cannot compel hospital to disclose name of potential bone marrow donor; *McFall* v. *Shimp*, 10 Pa. D. & C. 3d 90 (1978), court cannot compel a relative of person suffering from bone marrow disease to submit to a bone marrow transplant.

Blood donation or sale does not constitute a legal, medical, or ethical parallel. First, the selling of blood is not an open-market face-to-face transaction. We require medical organizations to act as the transfer agents. Some courts have even gone so far as to say the taking of blood plasma constitutes the practice of medicine; see *Mirsa, Inc.* v. *State Medical Board*, 42 Ohio St. 2d 399, 329 N.E. 2d 106 (1971). Second, the taking of only one pint of blood is not sufficiently life-threatening to the donor to be analogous to slavery or the taking of an organ.

19. More recently, some legislatures have required hospital personnel to ask for donations of body parts from relatives where no statement of intention to give has been made, if no donor card has been signed. See, e.g., N.Y. Public Health Law § 4351 (McKinney Supp. 1986). For an example of governmental initiatives in addressing transplantation issues, see *Final Report of the Task Force on Liver Transplantation in Massachusetts* (Fineberg Report) (May 1983).

20. Uniform Anatomical Gift Act § 6 (1987).

21. See, e.g., Pub. L. 99-509 § 9318. Citing a task force recommendation, the bill for the reconciliation of the 1987 budget amended the Social Security Act to require that hospitals, as a condition to receiving Medicare or Medicaid after October 1, 1987, establish written protocols "for the identification of potential organ donors that [make families] aware of the option of organ or tissue donation and their option to decline" (codified as 42 U.S.C.A. § 1320b-8(a) (West Supp. 1988)).

22. In 1984 Congress passed the National Organ Transplant Act, prohibiting the interstate sale of human organs (42 U.S.C.A. § 274(e) (West Supp. 1985)). California, Maryland, Michigan, New York, and Virginia also prohibit human organ sales. See "Regulating the Sale of Human Organs," *Virginia Law Review* 71, no. 6 (September 1985): 1023 n.84–85. Calabresi classifies such laws as rules which make an entitlement (here bodily organs) inalienable. A state may regulate an entitlement this way for paternalistic and/or distributional purposes. (Calabresi and Melamed, "Property Rules," pp. 1092–93, 1114–15, n. 50.)

23. Uniform Anatomical Gift Act § 10 (1987).

24. Intricate questions concerning the proving of claims, or the manner

in which the amount of monetary damages could be assessed, are not directly relevant to my hypothesis.

25. *In re Quinlan,* 70 N.J. 10, 355 A. 2d 647 (1976).

26. *In re Quinlan,* 137 N.J. Super. 227, 257–58 (Ch. Div. 1975), quoting *Schueler* v. *Strelinger,* 43 N.J. 330, 344, 204 A. 2d 577, 584 (1964).

27. *In re Quinlan,* 70 N.J. 10, 46, 355 A. 2d 647, 666–67.

28. *In re Quinlan,* 70 N.J. 10, 49, 355 A. 2d 647, 668.

29. If all persons involved in a decision to remove a respirator know they are accountable, the decision will only be made after intense collaboration with one another and deliberation over the patient's probable desires. See Robert A. Burt, *Taking Care of Strangers: The Rule of Law in Doctor-Patient Relations* (New York: Free Press, 1979), pp. 164–71.

30. See Burt, *Taking Care,* p. 152.

31. Burt sees the court as ultimately relieving the pain of Karen's observers, not of Karen herself. "The physicians had testified that Karen most likely perceived no pain while in her coma, even though it might seem otherwise to those who witnessed her reflexive grimaces and groans. . . . If she neither experienced pain in her coma nor would have any memory of suffering if she regained consciousness, avoiding pain would not be a reasonable ground for [removing her respirator]. But this pain, the only indisputable pain, was suffered by those around her—by family and friends, physicians and nurses—and not by her" (*Taking Care,* p. 151).

32. *Barber* v. *Superior Court,* 147 Cal. App. 3d 1006, 195 Cal. Rptr. 484 (1983). In this case, the defendants were charged with homicide for removing a respirator too quickly. The court held that the defendants could not be held criminally liable because there was not a clear duty to continue treatment in that particular case. Note, however, that criminal liability is based on an intentional wrong, not just on negligence.

33. The New Jersey Supreme Court decision in the Baby M case prompted much public debate and legislative (re)action (*In the Matter of Baby "M,"* 109 N.J. 396, 537 A. 2d 1227 (1988)). See, e.g., Larry Palmer, "No Rights for Sperm Donors," *New Jersey Law Journal,* 18 February 1988, p. 29. A New York commission has just recommended a ban on all surrogacy contracts. See *New York Times,* 26 June 1988, p. 1.

34. Donald A. Schön, *The Reflective Practitioner: How Professionals Think in Action* (New York: Basic Books, 1983), pp. 184–87.

35. *Howard* v. *Lecher,* 42 N.Y. 2d 109 (1977).

36. *Becker* v. *Schwartz,* 46 N.Y. 2d 401, 413–15, 413 N.Y.S. 2d 895, 901–02 (1978). In the companion case, Mrs. Park had previously given birth to an infant who died from polycystic kidney disease hours after its birth. She had been a patient of Dr. Chessin and his associates, all specialists in obstetrics, during her first pregnancy. When asked, Dr. Chessin informed Mr. and Mrs. Park that the disease was not hereditary, so there was little chance of their giving birth to a second child with the disease. Reassured,

Mrs. Park became pregnant again and gave birth to another child with polycystic kidney disease, who lived for only two and a half years. The disease *is* hereditary, in fact, and Mr. and Mrs. Park contended that had they known this they would never have conceived the second child. Like the Beckers, the Parks brought the lawsuit on their own behalf and that of their dead child. The court held consistently to the view that the child could not recover anything; the parents, however, were entitled to recover the amount of money already spent having to meet the medical needs of their child, but not for any emotional distress they might have suffered. In addition, the court asserted that damages could not put the infant in as good a position as she would have been in the absence of the alleged physician negligence, since the court felt unable to place a value on the state of never having been born.

37. *Becker* v. *Schwartz,* 46 N.Y. 2d 401, 411–412, 413 N.Y.S. 2d 895, 900–901 (1978).

38. *Berman* v. *Allan,* 80 N.J. 421, 428–30, 404 A. 2d 8, 12–13 (1979).

39. Fowler V. Harper and Fleming James, *The Law of Torts,* vol. 2 (Boston: Little, Brown & Co., 1956), § 12.1, 12.4. We can take the more modern position of "economic analysis" to arrive at the same result, although some notions of "fault" are at play by the time we reach *Becker* v. *Schwartz.*

40. The court considered the case of *Gleitman* v. *Cosgrove,* 49 N.J. 22 (1967).

41. "One of the most deeply held beliefs of our society is that life— whether experienced with or without a major physical handicap—is more precious than non-life" (*Berman* v. *Allan,* 80 N.J. 421, 429, 404 A. 2d 8, 12).

42. Judge Cooke would base Mrs. Howard's recovery on the physician-patient relationship, in which the physician's failure to inform prevented Mrs. Howard from terminating her pregnancy. "Certain facts of life of the 1970's must be recognized and accepted at the outset. One such fact is the legal right of a mother to abort a pregnancy (*Roe* v. *Wade,* 410 U.S. 113; Penal Law, § 125.05). Another is the development and application of tests to identify carriers of Tay-Sachs disease and the occurrence of that disease in their yet unborn offspring. . . . With the information from this fatal disease, parents could make an informed, although difficult, decision as to whether to continue or to terminate the pregnancy" (*Howard* v. *Lecher,* 42 N.Y. 2d 109, 113-15, 397 N.Y.S. 2d 362, 366 (Cooke, J., dissenting)). The father, however, has no parallel claim. Though Dr. Lecher's malpractice may cause Mr. Howard to suffer as much as his wife, Mr. Howard stands outside the sphere of duty of the physician-patient relationship. (*Howard* v. *Lecher,* 42 N.Y. 2d 109, 116, 397 N.Y.S. 2d 363, 368.)

43. In *Doe* v. *Bolton,* the Supreme Court struck down provisions of a Georgia abortion statute which required advance approval by an abortion

committee made up of hospital staff, as well as confirmation by two additional physicians. However, the Court upheld a provision that allows a hospital to refuse to admit a patient for an abortion. (410 U.S. 179, 195–99 (1973).)

44. Individuals who are of childbearing age and contemplating children have intense interest in the growing knowledge of prenatal detection of genetic disorders. In general, potential parents have an episodic rather than a scientific interest in genetic knowledge. As the childbearing years pass, their knowledge is not likely to be current, even assuming it was ever accurate. In addition, there is a large number of people of childbearing age who do not have any knowledge of genetic disorders for a variety of reasons. Nevertheless, access to this knowledge is an important health-enhancing resource from the perspective of the parents.

45. *Berman* v. *Allan*, 80 N.J. 421, 440, 404 A. 2d 8, 18 (Handler, J., concurring).

46. "The injury consists of a diminished childhood in being born of parents kept ignorant of her defective state while unborn and who, on that account, were less fit to accept and assume their parental responsibilities. The frightful weight of the child's natural handicap has been made more burdensome by defendants' negligence because her parents' capacity has been impaired" (*Berman* v. *Allan*, 80 N.J. 421, 442, 404 A. 2d 8, 19 (Handler, J., concurring)).

47. Since the meaning of an experience to an individual depends on countless internal and external variables, it may have a favorable impact on Person A, no impact on Person B, and an impact contrary to that sought on Person C; see Joseph Goldstein, "Psychoanalysis and Jurisprudence," *Yale Law Journal* 77 (1968): 1071–72.

48. "There must be a way to free physicians, in the pursuit of their healing vocation, from possible contamination by self-interest or self-protection concerns which would inhibit their independent medical judgments for the well-being of their dying patients" (*In re Quinlan*, 70 N.J. 10, 49, 355 A. 2d 647, 668 (1976)). Defensive medicine has been divided into two categories: positive, where physicians prescribe unnecessary tests and treatments, and negative, where physicians refrain from high-risk treatments and innovative procedures or refuse to take patients with complicated problems. Positive defensive medicine may increase the quality of care while decreasing the quantity. Negative defensive medicine may decrease both the quality and the quantity of medical care. The correlation between medical malpractice liability and the occurrence of defensive medicine is still sketchy. However, one study shows positive defensive medicine occurs more frequently in states with a high malpractice threat than in states with a low threat. (Project, "The Medical Malpractice Threat: A Study of Defensive Medicine," *Duke Law Journal* (1971): 939, 948–49, 956.)

49. *Schloendorff* v. *New York Hospital*, 211 N.Y. 125, 129, 105 N.E. 92,

93 (1914). This case is looked upon and cited as the wellspring of informed consent. See *Lambert* v. *Park,* 597 F. 2d 236, 237 (10th Cir. 1979); *Henderson* v. *Milobsky,* 595 F. 2d 654, 657 (D.C. Cir. 1978); *In re Storar,* 52 N.Y. 2d 363, 376, 438 N.Y.S. 2d 266, 272 (1981). We should bear in mind that *Schloendorff* was in fact a case of "assault" in which the physician was held legally liable for an unauthorized operation, not a case of a negligently performed operation. The operational rules for assault and negligence are different, but the doctrine of informed consent as developed for malpractice cases is a hybrid of these two legal doctrines.

50. "The common law's vision of informed consent is confusing and confused. Its frequently articulated underlying purpose—to promote patients' decisional authority over their medical fate—has been severely compromised from the beginning. The wish that patients can or should be allowed to make their own decisions, based on the fullest disclosure possible, runs through most of the opinions. But once the wish has been given its separate due, the rest of the opinion ignores that dream and instead defers to those realities of legal, medical, and human life which are opposed to fostering patients' decision-making. Thus the doctrine of informed consent remains a symbol which despite widespread currency has had little impact on patients' decision-making, either in legal theory or medical practice" (Jay Katz, "Informed Consent—A Fairy Tale? Law's Vision," *University of Pittsburgh Law Review* 39, no. 2 [Winter 1977]: 137, 139). See also Jay Katz, *The Silent World of Doctor and Patient* (New York: Free Press, 1984), pp. 48–84.

51. By looking at other models, we realize that too much of our public discussion of medicine has been dominated by a biomedical model of disease. But being under medical care does not necessarily mean a person is socially dysfunctional. The kidney patient using home dialysis has a disease, for instance, although he is not necessarily "sick" from a social perspective. The prevailing biomedical model also does not account for such conditions as diabetes or schizophrenia. Even with the biomedical imbalances of both diseases, many afflicted individuals function successfully in society. In addition, a biomedical model tends to exclude a full analysis of such phenomena as "pain," reducing them to specific physiological functions to be dealt with by medication or surgery. In some instances the refusal of the "patient" to assume the passive "sick" role by wanting to participate in the management of his or her diabetes has caused many physicians to resist new techniques of managing this condition. Or even more significant occurrences for modern medicine are many patients undertaking "self-care" and not following their doctors' directions about medication. A sick-role analysis of disease does not permit us to think about defining an appropriate place for modern medicine in a society becoming older and thus containing increasingly more disabled individuals. See Talcott Parsons, "The Sick Role and the Role of

the Physician Reconsidered," *Health and Society* 53, no. 3 (Summer 1975): 257.

52. George L. Engel, "The Need for a New Medical Model: A Challenge for Biomedicine," *Science,* 8 April 1977, p. 130.

53. In England there is no doctrine of informed consent separate from the idea of ordinary standards of care (*Sidaway* v. *Board of Governors of the Bethlem Royal Hospital,* 2 W.L.R. 480 (1985)).

54. *Canturbury* v. *Spence,* 464 F. 2d 772 (D.C. Cir. 1972).

55. One consequence of highly specialized medicine and its accompanying system of referrals is that physicians are no longer dependent on their reputations among patients but upon the referrals from their fellow physicians (Theodore J. Schneyer, "Informed Consent and the Danger of Bias in the Formation of Medical Disclosure Practices," *Wisconsin Law Review* (1976): 137–38).

56. *Karp* v. *Cooley,* 493 F. 2d 408, 412 n.4 (5th Cir. 1974).

57. *Karp* v. *Cooley,* 493 F. 2d 408.

58. There are many curious features about this case—the unwillingness of Dr. Michael De Bakey, another world-famous heart surgeon who was also trying to develop an artificial heart pump, to testify as an expert witness on behalf of Mrs. Karp, for example—that need not detain us here. See Thomas Thompson, *Hearts: Of Surgeons and Transplants, Miracles and Disasters Along the Cardiac Frontier* (Greenwich, Conn.: Fawcett Publications, 1971).

59. When Dr. Cooley performed Mr. Karp's operation in 1969, he was one of the few surgeons in the world doing heart transplantation. Despite the public clamor that accompanied the early heart transplants, the operations were relatively unsuccessful from the patients' perspective; their survival rate as a whole was quite low. On the day of the Karp operation in 1969, only three of Cooley's previous nineteen transplant patients remained alive. At best, heart transplantation was then a last-resort treatment and at worst an "experimental" procedure that prolonged life for only a very short time. Since the artificial pump had never been used in a human, it was an experimental device by almost any account. See Thompson, *Hearts,* pp. 153–243. With the development of antirejection drugs in the past few years, especially cyclosporine, heart transplants are now being done around the country. The one-year survival rate is about 80 percent. ("Renaissance in Organ Transplants," *Editorial Research Reports,* 8 July 1983, p. 495.) The federal government regulates the use of medical devices under the Federal Food, Drug and Cosmetic Act. See Medical Devices Amendment of 1976, 21 U.S.C.A. § 360(c) (West Supp. 1988).

60. The point is made in Thompson, *Hearts.*

61. Thompson, *Hearts,* pp. 227–35.

62. *Karp* v. *Cooley,* 493 F. 2d 408, 416 n.6.

63. William C. DeVries et al., "Clinical Use of the Total Artificial Heart," *New England Journal of Medicine* 310, no. 5 (February 1984): 273.

64. Pierre M. Galletti, "Replacement of the Heart with a Mechanical Device: The Case of Dr. Barney Clark," *New England Journal of Medicine* 310, no. 5 (February 1984): 312.

Chapter 2: Hospitals, Mental Hospitals, and Other Caretaking Institutions

1. Chester M. Southam, "Homotransplantation of Human Cell Lines," *Science,* January 25, 1957, p. 158.

2. This case has also been discussed in Jay Katz, *Experimentation with Human Beings* (New York: Russell Sage Foundation, 1972), pp. 1–65; and Joseph Goldstein et al., *Criminal Law: Theory and Process,* 2nd ed. (New York: Free Press, 1974), pp. 81–86.

3. Dr. Southam did mention that signed permission forms were, in fact, used with Ohio State Penitentiary prisoners who participated in these previous experiments, but that this practice was due to "the law-oriented personalities of these men, rather than for any medical reason" (Letter from Dr. Chester Southam to Dr. Edward Mandel, dated 5 July 1963 in Katz, *Experimentation,* p. 11).

4. Dr. Rosenfeld, coordinator of medicine for the hospital's Blumberg Pavilion, had eighteen patients in his ward who were injected, without his knowledge, with the live cancer suspension. Dr. Custodio, who performed most of these injections, officially served under Dr. Rosenfeld. (Katz, *Experimentation,* p. 15.)

5. Mr. Hyman, who was also a lawyer, chose to represent himself in this case. In presenting the facts to the court, he did not seek to have the judges explicitly determine the legality of the experiment. Rather, he asked the court to compel the hospital to turn the medical records of the twenty-two patients involved in the experiment over to him. He argued that as a director of the hospital he had a duty to determine whether they could be subject to civil or criminal liability. (Note that his emphasis was not placed on representing the patients' personal interests, which might have invoked the doctor-patient privilege impediment to his receiving the files.) In support of the gravity of his request, Mr. Hyman referred to the resignations of three physicians, the "large amount of money" the federal government had paid to support the experiment, and, most notably, the medical principles established at Nuremberg, in which several Nazi doctors were hanged for their failure to obtain informed consent from experimental subjects. In further support of his legal right to review, he went on to characterize the hospital board of directors' overwhelming majority acceptance of the report of the Medical Grievance Committee as a "whitewash." (Katz, *Experimentation,* pp. 19, 41–44.)

6. *In the Matter of Hyman v. Jewish Chronic Disease Hospital,* 15 N.Y. 2d 317, 323, 206 N.E. 2d 338, 339 (1965).

7. It is also instructive to note that this 1963 view of clinical research in a hospital did not focus on the issue of "informed consent" in the same way the organization does currently. Despite the controversy concerning what the patients were actually told before the injection, the research team and Dr. Mandel, their new collaborator, were very candid; it is clear that the patients were not to be told that the injection contained live cancer cells for fear of "unnecessary anxieties, disturbances, or phobias." (Affidavit of Dr. Custodio, in Katz, *Experimentation,* p. 25.) The research team maintained that they did obtain the oral consent of the patients for a test of their immunological responses, while their challengers asserted that even if this much was true, it was not made clear to the patient that the test was unrelated to his or her own treatment.

8. The 1930s saw the advent of medical specialization, which offered an attractive alternative for medical students to the standard general practice. This modernization was linked to the ultimate demise of house calls as physicians became more hospital-centered by necessity in their various, more technical fields. See generally, Paul Starr, *The Social Transformation of American Medicine* (New York: Basic Books, 1982), and Lewis Thomas, *The Youngest Science: Notes of a Medicine-Watcher* (New York: Viking Press, 1983).

9. Fundamental to these questions is the definition of medicine itself. The court could have seen that it was the organizational purpose of hospitals that was actually being brought into question, revolving around some large and complex notion of medicine, much as it is fair to say a lawsuit against General Motors involves the nature of manufacturing. Had the litigation involved General Motors, it would have been necessary for the court to determine whether the concern was over the portion of the organization that produces refrigerators or engines for buses. When looking at hospitals, however, we do not ordinarily ask such categorical questions. Our cultural ethos favoring healing rarely permits such hard, analytical questions to be asked about the healing institutions we have organized—even by judges. For an analysis of our evolving concepts of organizations and institutions in general, see Gareth Morgan, *Images of Organization* (Beverly Hills, Calif.: Sage Publications, 1986).

10. To the degree that individual professionals within hospitals feel constrained by "review committees" and other mechanisms that have since been put into place to protect human subjects, that frustration must be offset by realizing the historically proven necessity of those mechanisms. From the larger perspective of modern hospitals with recognized multifunctions, individual constraints serve to oversee and therefore legitimize each function they address. This legitimacy has led to a burgeoning field of biomedical research, which is indoctrinated even in early medical training. The

most prestigious positions within the medical profession are those involving research and teaching. Such nonpecuniary reward incentives tend to emphasize the physician-scientist role. In the Jewish Chronic Disease case, it was apparent that just the opportunity to be associated with Dr. Southam, who was at the apex of the significant professional hierarchy as physician scientist, represented professional advancement potential.

11. For insightful analysis of the modern relationship between doctor and patient, see generally, Jay Katz, *The Silent World of Doctor and Patient* (New York: Free Press, 1984); Robert A. Burt, *Taking Care of Strangers: The Rule of Law in Doctor-Patient Relations* (New York: Free Press, 1979), pp. 92–173; and William F. May, *The Physician's Covenant: Images of the Healer in Medical Ethics* (Philadelphia: Westminster Press, 1983).

12. The sanctioning of Dr. Southam was important not so much because he and his colleague knew that they were, to some extent, deceiving the patients, but because it was necessary to set a standard for doctor-patient transactions in the context of allopathic medicine (in which a second condition is produced in the patient because it is incompatible with or antagonistic to the first).

13. 45 C.F.R. 46.116 (1973).

14. Marilyn T. Baker and Harvey A. Taub, "Readability of Informed Consent Forms for Research in a Veterans Administration Medical Center," *Journal of the American Medical Association,* 250, no. 19 (November 1983): 2646–48.

15. Katz, *The Silent World,* p. 85.

16. Katz spoke of the undeniable realities of hospital life, despite courtroom pronouncements of self-determination. "The rule of law in hospitals continued to be guided by principles of custody, not liberty" (ibid., p. 59).

17. Although psychiatry and psychoanalysis are often confused, it is important to note that we are dealing with psychiatry, a medical specialty, and not psychoanalysis, a theory of human behavior. These researchers assumed there was more than a psychodynamic explanation for human behavior—that possibly there were biomedical causes, which in some cases could be subject to manipulation by the techniques of modern medical practice. They were primarily concerned with those persons whose aggressiveness had led to social sanctioning in the form of incarceration in either prisons or state mental hospitals. They were, at one level, seeking to bring the benefits of modern medical science to a group of patients who are basically shunned by both society and most members of the medical profession. Note that their hypothesis demonstrated the pragmatism of medicine by posing the question in this poignant social form rather than in the abstract form of What is the relationship of the human brain to human behavior?

18. *Kaimowitz* v. *Michigan Department of Mental Health,* Prison Law Reporter 2 (1973): 433. Gabe Kaimowitz, as a member of the Medical

Committee for Human Rights in Michigan, sued on behalf of certain individual members of that committee and at least twenty-four involuntarily
committed patients.

19. *Kaimowitz,* Appendix Item no. 1.

20. Psychosurgery was defined before a Senate Subcommittee on Health
in 1973 as "a surgical removal or destruction of brain tissue or the cutting
of brain tissue to disconnect one part of the brain from another, with the
intent of altering the behavior, even though there may be no direct evidence
of structural disease or damage to the brain" (Testimony of Dr. Bertram
S. Brown, Director of the National Institute of Mental Health, U.S., Congress, Senate, Subcommittee on Health of the Committee of Labor and
Public Welfare, *Quality of Health Care—Human Experimentation,* 93rd
Cong., 1st sess., 23 February 1973, p. 339).

21. Vernon Mark and Frank Ervin, *Violence and the Brain* (New York:
Harper & Row, 1970). It should be noted here that Dr. Mark, upon learning
of the researchers' project from Dr. Rodin, objected strenuously on ethical
grounds. His own psychosurgical research had used only epileptic patients.
He told Dr. Rodin he felt strongly that they had no right to make lesions
in a "healthy" brain when the individual suffered from rage attacks only.
See also Vernon Mark, "Social and Ethical Issues: Brain Surgery in Aggressive Epileptics," *Hastings Center Report* 3, no. 1 (February 1973): 1.

22. Several years later the National Commission for the Protection of
Human Subjects of Biomedical and Behavioral Research examined all of the
available evidence on psychosurgery and concluded, contrary to the *Kaimowitz* court, that the procedure could be performed on detained persons,
provided a set of elaborate safeguards was followed. One commissioner
argued against distinguishing detained persons from those who voluntarily
committed themselves, arguing that both types should be dealt with similarly and recognizing the realities of the "last resort" position of just being
in the mental hospital for any significant period of time.

23. Professors Robert Burt and Francis Allen, the court-appointed coun-
sel and co-counsel for the intended patient, argued that, given the extreme
risks and uncertainties of modern psychosurgery, it would be "cruel and
unusual punishment" to compel that surgery on an involuntarily committed
patient, thus violating the Constitution's Eighth Amendment protection.
Moreover, the attorneys argued, the patient's subsequent withdrawal of
consent to the surgical experiment after being released from the institution
by the court (on other grounds) and his testimony indicated that his initial
consent had actually been based on a desire to be considered a "cooperative" patient and hopefully obtain his release as a result. The attorneys
concluded: "Institutional confinement is itself so inherently coercive that
the taint of state compulsion cannot be adequately dispelled to satisfy the
necessary burden of showing consent." (Robert A. Burt and Francis Allen,
"At the Present Time Experimental Neurosurgery Cannot be Performed on

Involuntarily Confined Mental Patients," *Law Quadrangle Notes of the University of Michigan* 18 [Fall 1973]: 9, 11.) Note that the authors limit their conclusions to "the present time," leaving room for medical advancements that could make neurosurgery "widely accepted conventional therapy for aggressive conduct" and thus no longer require special consent (p. 15).

24. While there are short-term psychiatry wards in regular hospitals, these are probably attempts to return the patients to society, whereas a mental hospital is not a place from which people generally return.

25. Dr. Thomas Szasz argues that the very notion of mental illness is a myth purveyed only to enforce conformity and that this myth is only tolerable, if at all, when each individual accepts the mental illness label. Accordingly, he argues, civil commitment laws cannot be reformed but must be abolished, since they rest on the unacceptable premise that one person can define another as mentally ill without the other's consent. See Thomas Szasz, *Psychiatric Slavery* (New York: Free Press, 1977); then note Burt's critique in *Taking Care of Strangers,* p. 43.

26. *Superintendent of Belchertown State School* v. *Saikewicz,* 370 N.E. 2d 417 (1977). It should be noted that while many parents provide ample accounts of children at this age who could communicate and even verbally express themselves to strangers to some extent, Mr. Saikewicz's profound retardation was said to have made meaningful communication with him impossible.

27. As pointed out by Burt, the only indisputable "pain" involved with a "silent patient," whether he or she is comatose or profoundly retarded, is the anguish felt by those around the patient. Beyond that, actually feeling or understanding pain, and even hypothetically making choices in that regard, remains an uncertainty. I want to take this opportunity to express my sincere debt and appreciation to Robert Burt for his "silent patient" analysis.

28. The *Saikewicz* court explained, "In this case, a ward of a state institution was discovered to have an invariably fatal illness, the only effective—in the sense of life-prolonging—treatment for which involved serious and painful intrusions on the patient's body. While an emergency existed with regard to taking action to begin treatment, it was not a case in which immediate action was required. Nor was this a case in which life-saving, as distinguished from life-prolonging, procedures were available. Because the individual involved was thought to be incompetent to make necessary decisions, the officials of the State institutions properly initiated proceedings in the Probate Court" (370 N.E. 2d 417, 433 (1977)).

29. In footnote 4 of the opinion, the court adds that the probate court's decision was acceptable, given that the report calling into question the evidence regarding the lower success rate of chemotherapy with older pa-

tients was not before the court (*Superintendent of Belchertown State School* v. *Saikewicz,* 370 N.E. 2d 417, 421 (1977)).

30. Joseph Saikewicz died within four months of the commencement of the litigation of a complication of his leukemia, bronchial pneumonia. In the court's view, he died without "pain or discomfort," although as laypersons we may question this conclusion since the court earlier stated that he could not communicate or understand pain.

31. *Halderman* v. *Pennhurst State School and Hospital,* 446 F.Supp. 1295, 1308 (1977) *aff'd in part* and *rev'd in part,* 612 F. 2d 84 (CA3 1979), *rev'd,* 451 U.S. 1 (1981).

32. *In the Matter of Hofbauer,* 47 N.Y. 2d 648, 657 (1979).

33. This is a curious position to take from conventional medicine's perspective, since the longer one waits to commence chemotherapy the less likely it is that the therapy will be successful.

34. *New York Times,* 18 July 1980, sec. 4, p. 5.

35. It is important to note that, except when dealing with surgical treatments, cancer "cures" are generally talked about in terms of survival rates for an extended number of years.

36. *In the Matter of Hofbauer,* 47 N.Y. 2d 648, 656 (1979).

37. Their personal, even religious, views may have allowed them to accept their son's death in a manner different from our own—a point I will come back to later in this book.

38. In 1988 a judge in Tioga County, New York, ordered that a four-year-old leukemia patient must continue with chemotherapy, despite his parents' objection to the treatment. The parents objected to the toxicity of the chemotherapy drugs and feared that the long-term effects are not known. They chose nutritional therapy as a safer form of treatment for their son. The judge based his decision on *Hofbauer,* noting that in the present case, no other doctor would recommend the alternative treatment preferred by the parents. In his decision, the judge called the parents (the father is a local chiropractor) "extremely intelligent, well-educated, conscientious, and loving parents" who were nevertheless insufficiently qualified, as determined by New York State law, to make medical decisions for a dangerously ill child. (*Binghamton Press & Sun-Bulletin,* 25 May 1988, p. 1.)

39. *Weber* v. *Stony Brook Hospital,* 60 N.Y. 2d 208, 456 N.E. 2d 1186 (1983); *United States* v. *University Hospital, State University of New York at Stony Brook,* 729 F. 2d 144 (2d Cir., 1984). The first state supreme court case on this point came when the federal Department of Health and Human Services (DHHS) sought to enforce treatment of defective newborns after the national publicity centering around the Bloomington, Indiana, Baby Doe case, *In re Infant Doe,* No. GU8204-004A (Monroe County Cir. Ct., 12 April 1982), *writ of mandamus dismissed sub nom. State ex rel Infant*

Doe v. *Baker,* No. 482 section 140 (Ind. Sup. Ct., 27 May 1982), *cert. denied Infant Doe* v. *Bloomington Hospital,* 464 U.S. 961, 104 S. Ct. 394 (1983). The DHHS used section 504 of the Rehabilitation Act of 1973, which made it illegally discriminatory to deny benefits from a federally funded program to an otherwise-qualified handicapped individual, 29 U.S.C. § 794 (1982). The rule called for large nondiscrimination signs to be posted in federally funded hospital nurseries stating that all "medically beneficial" treatments were required and not to be denied due to handicap, as well as a toll-free Handicapped Infant Hotline number to encourage anonymous reports to federal authorities regarding suspected denials of food or "customary care." The American Academy of Pediatrics and other medical groups quickly challenged the regulation in federal court, whereupon it was invalidated on the ground that, in promulgating it, the DHHS had ignored various require-ments of the Administrative Procedure Act, especially those for notice and comment by interested parties (*American Academy of Pediatrics* v. *Heckler,* 561 F.Supp. 395, 398–401 (D.D.C., 1983)). DHHS recurred the effort with its final rule, 45 C.F.R. § 84.55 (1985), which dispensed with the procedural objections to its predecessor. The rule called for the conspicuous nondis-crimination signs but with the addition that "reasonable medical judgments in selecting among alternative courses of treatment will be respected." The signs also were to include the Handicapped Infant Hotline number. This final regulation was recently rejected by the U.S. Supreme Court, *Bowen* v. *American Hospital Association,* 476 U.S. 610, 106 S. Ct. 2101 (1986). The *Bowen* court held that a defective newborn whose parents have not author-ized consent or treatment is not being discriminatorily denied of anything by the hospitals and is therefore not subject to section 504 of the Federal Rehabilitation Act. Without the parents' consent, the infant is neither "otherwise qualified" for treatment nor has he been denied care "solely by reason of his handicap." The court criticized and rejected federal interven-tion in such personal and state matters, stating, "Section 504 does not authorize the [DHHS] Secretary to give unsolicited advice either to parents, to hospitals, or to state officials who are faced with difficult treatment decisions concerning handicapped children" (476 U.S. 610, 647).

40. The presidential commission also recommends ultimate responsi-bility in the parents, with professional support by the attending physicians and medical institution. See U.S. President's Commission for the Study of Ethical Problems in Medicine and Biomedical and Behavioral Research, *Deciding to Forgo Life-Sustaining Treatment* (Washington, D.C.: U.S. Gov-ernment Printing Office, 1983). Burt, however, rejects the commission's stance as anticommunal and argues against isolating decision-making au-thority in parents. He defines "true physicians" and "true parents" as always attempting to save the life of the threatened child. See Robert A. Burt, "The Ideal of Community in the Work of the President's Commis-sion," *Cardozo Law Review* 6 (Winter 1984): 267.

41. *Estelle* v. *Gamble,* 429 U.S. 1066, 97 S. Ct. 798 (1976) held that Eighth Amendment protection against cruel and unusual punishment "establishes the government's obligation to provide medical care for those whom it is punishing by incarceration."

42. *Commissioner of Correction* v. *Myers,* 379 Mass. 255 (1979), 399 N.E. 2d 452.

43. I say "apparently" because of Professor Burt's *Kaimowitz* analysis which calls into question the prisoner's stated goal. He may have felt that by refusing consent to his jailers his life came to have more significance to them or himself. There is also the element of a desire for "self-rule," amid the involuntary incarceration, that Professor Burt discusses in his book (*Taking Care of Strangers,* pp. 1–21).

44. The attending physician, Tai Jin Chung, admitted to the court that he had never administered dialysis to an unwilling patient or heard of others doing so and that it was not possible to use a general anesthetic to subdue a patient. He also testified that in the unlikely but conceivable event that the patient's struggling dislodged one of the needles connected to his arm, three to four minutes' loss of blood could prove fatal. (*Myers,* 379 Mass. 255, 259, 399 N.E. 2d 452, 454.)

45. See discussion of federal funding for kidney dialysis in chapter 1.

46. Note that, in general, states do allow force-feeding of state penitentiary prisoners engaged in political "hunger strikes." See *In re Caulk,* 480 A. 2d 93 (1984), from New Hampshire; *Von Holden* v. *Chapman,* 87 A.D. 2d 66, 450 N.Y.S. 2d 623 (1982); and *White* v. *Narick,* 292 S.E. 2d 54 (1982), a West Virginia case; but cf. *Zant* v. *Prevatte,* 248 Ga. 832, 286 S.E. 2d 715 (1982).

47. "There comes a time when physicians, family, and friends must cease their efforts to fight death, not in order to abandon the patient, but to provide care and only care. More aggressive treatment under some conditions misses the mark and ultimately neglects the patient" (May, *Physician's Covenant,* p. 79).

48. See Burt, *Taking Care of Strangers,* ch. 7, "Conversation with Silent Patients," pp. 144–73.

49. May, *Physician's Covenant,* pp. 74–77.

50. A large amount of evidence (which I will not review here) led to the conclusion that "treatment" for mental illness and perhaps mental retardation is best done somewhere other than in the present kinds of institutions that these two areas are centered in currently. Anyone who has visited one of these facilities could easily feel that there must be a better way of healing. But what is curious is our inability to develop those better means.

51. "From Country Asylums to City Streets: The Contradiction Between Deinstitutionalization and State Mental Health Funding Priorities—Report of Council President Carol Bellamy" (New York: New York City Council, 1979).

52. The case of *Rivers* v. *Katz,* 67 N.Y. 2d 485, 495 N.E. 2d 337 (1986), has seemingly begun the clarification process. Rivers held that the mere fact that patients are mentally ill, or even involuntarily committed, does not alone constitute "a sufficient basis to conclude that they lack the mental capacity to comprehend the consequences of their decision to refuse medication that poses a significant risk to their physical well-being" (*Rivers,* 67 N.Y. 2d 485, 494). The court declared that these patients retain their "liberty interest in avoiding the unwanted administration of antipsychotic medication," save for emergency compelling state interests (*Rivers,* 67 N.Y. 2d 485, 495).

53. A person involuntarily committed to a state institution for the mentally retarded was held to have constitutionally protected liberty interests under the due process clause of the Fourteenth Amendment to reasonably safe conditions of confinement, freedom from unreasonable bodily restraints, and such minimally adequate training as reasonably might be required by these interests (*Youngberg* v. *Romeo,* 457 U.S. 307, 102 S. Ct. 2452 (1982)).

54. *Klostermann* v. *Cuomo,* 61 N.Y. 2d 525; 463 N.E. 2d 588; 475 N.Y.S. 2d 247 (1984).

55. See Joseph Goldstein, Anna Freud, and Albert J. Solnit, *Before the Best Interests of the Child* (New York: Free Press, 1979), pp. 49–50.

Chapter 3: Specialization and the Physician's Social Obligations

1. Even the "family practitioner" of today is actually a specialist in referring the patient to other specialists. See William F. May, *The Physician's Covenant: Images of the Healer in Medical Ethics* (Philadelphia: Westminster Press, 1983), pp. 37–38.

2. Ignorance of an injury's origin is a more widespread and serious problem than is normally assumed. In the Quinlan case, for instance, the inability of anyone to tell the doctors what might have led to her coma— drugs or a blow to the head, for example—created some of the medical uncertainty of her case and made it *sui generis.*

3. *Landeros* v. *Flood,* 17 Cal. 3d 399, 406, 551 P. 2d 389, 391, 131 Cal. Rptr. 69, 71 (1976).

4. C. Henry Kempe et al., "The Battered-Child Syndrome," *Journal of the American Medical Association,* 181, no. 1 (7 July 1962): 17–24.

5. The physician should assume that if the child has some readily identifiable symptoms of intentional injury, the person who inflicted those injuries may have also inflicted other indiscernible injuries. Thus, the physician should do a more in-depth diagnosis including, perhaps, a complete x-ray examination. In the case described above, had the physician ordered an x-ray examination, he would have discovered a fracture on the infant's skull. A correctly diagnosed case of the battered child syndrome means that

all the pathological conditions, including the hidden skull injuries, would receive appropriate medical and surgical attention. See *Landeros* v. *Flood,* at 406, 551 P. 2d at 391, 131 Cal. Rptr. at 71.

6. Kempe et al., "The Battered-Child Syndrome," p. 20.

7. See, e.g., California Penal Code §§ 11165–72 (West Supp. 1986).

8. *Landeros,* 17 Cal. 3d 399, 551 P. 2d 389, 131 Cal. Rptr. 69.

9. Joseph Goldstein, Anna Freud, and Albert J. Solnit, *Before the Best Interests of the Child* (New York: Free Press, 1979), pp. 73, 87.

10. Ibid., pp. 85–86.

11. See Robert A. Burt, *Taking Care of Strangers: The Rule of Law in Doctor-Patient Relations* (New York: Free Press, 1979), ch. 3.

12. A. D. Woozley, "A Duty to Rescue: Some Thoughts on Criminal Liability," *Virginia Law Review* 69 (1983): 1273. The author considers why a legal requirement of a duty to rescue runs counter to the American common-law tradition. He notes that there seems to be "a deep-seated and widespread attitude that the choice [to rescue] . . . somebody to whom one has no relationship . . . should be left to the individual as a moral choice, in which the law should not interfere" (p. 1275).

13. *United States* v. *University Hosp., State Univ. of New York at Stony Brook,* 729 F. 2d 144 (2d Cir. 1984).

14. Note that the entire litigation, in both the state and federal courts, was directed toward the hospital rather than individual physicians. See *Weber* v. *Stony Brook Hospital,* 60 N.Y. 2d 208, 456 N.E. 2d 1186 (1983).

15. *United States* v. *University Hospital,* 729 F. 2d 144, 160.

16. Growing medical capacities bring about a form of cultural transformation, requiring a redefinition of social duty and thus a rethinking of law's ability to impose social obligations.

17. This lack of certainty in law's definition of the social duty is an important check on parental and medical decision-making. No conscientious lawyer could assure the hospital, the physicians, or the parents that a jury would never convict them of the crime of homicide, but any advice given would provide the social background against which a decision about treatment would be made. The uncertainty of law reminds those involved that the "preservation of life and health" has a variety of definitions and that opposing views ought to be carefully considered.

18. For an in-depth look at treatment decisions concerning severely impaired infants made over a two-and-a-half-year period at the Yale–New Haven Hospital, see Raymond S. Duff and A. G. M. Campbell, "Moral and Ethical Dilemmas in the Special-Care Nursery," *New England Journal of Medicine* 289, no. 17 (October 1973): 890.

19. *Tarasoff* v. *Regents of Univ. of Cal.,* 17 Cal. 3d 425, 551 P. 2d 334, 131 Cal. Rptr. 14 (1976).

20. Id., at 441–42, 551 P. 2d at 347, 131 Cal. Rptr. at 27.

21. Before adopting such facile reasoning, the court should have consid-

ered the differences between psychotherapists and most physicians, especially psychiatrists. Most psychiatrists do practice some form of psychotherapy, but the vast majority specialize in psychotrophic drug treatment, not psychotherapy. Furthermore, psychiatrists are committed to medicine's biomedical model of disease rather than the psychotherapists' biopsychosocial model which views the patient's problem as a function of biological, psychological, and social phenomena. When a court imposes the psychiatrist-biomedical framework on a psychotherapist, it automatically limits the social obligations of the nonmedically trained psychotherapist. (George L. Engel, "The Need for a New Medical Model: A Challenge for Biomedicine," *Science,* 8 April 1977, pp. 129, 134.)

22. I do not recognize a distinction between voluntary and involuntary commitment, since I believe that the social fabric is implicitly coercive in either case. Law itself has blurred any distinction. Parents may commit their children to institutions solely for the purpose of treatment. While some may be able to argue that this action is voluntary on the parents' part, no one can say that the particular child is volunteering for commitment. See, e.g., *Parham* v. *J.R.,* 442 U.S. 584, 99 S. Ct. 2493 (1979).

23. Under California Welfare & Institutions Code § 5251 (West 1984), a physician or psychologist with at least five years' experience has the authority to commit a patient.

24. *Bellah* v. *Greenson,* 81 Cal. App. 3d 614, 146 Cal. Rptr. 535 (1978) (failure to take appropriate measures to prevent a patient's self-harm is a breach of duty, but there is no duty to disclose unless the patient is threatening to others); *Stepakoff* v. *Kantar,* 473 N.E. 2d 1131 (Mass. 1985) (no specific legal duty to safeguard suicidal patient beyond the duty to exercise the care and skill customarily exercised by an average qualified psychiatrist).

25. Most of this factual description comes from Berton Roueché, "Annals of Medicine," *The New Yorker,* 9 September 1978, pp. 84–100, but I have added some other facts about referrals. I have also assumed that everyone is basically a good psychiatrist and that hospitals are good ones.

26. Electroconvulsive therapy should not be confused with electric shock treatment, which is applied as a form of behavior modification (Comment, "Recent Developments in Behavior Modification," *Nebraska Law Review* 60, no. 2 (1981): 363, 397).

27. This means that when her private insurance and other financial means are exhausted, she might be forced to spend the remainder of her life in a public mental hospital, possibly a large state-run facility. Medicare/ Medicaid will only reimburse up to $312.50 with respect to expenses incurred in any calendar year in connection with the treatment of mental, psychoneurotic, or personality disorders of an individual who is not an inpatient at the time such expenses are incurred (42 U.S.C.A. § 13951(c) (West 1983)).

28. I am especially indebted to my colleague H. Richard Beresford for my understanding of ECT, which I gained while team-teaching and developing materials for a Law and Medicine course at Cornell Law School with him. For a recent summary of the effectiveness of ECT, see "Electroconvulsive Therapy—Consensus Conference," *Journal of the American Medical Association* 254, no. 15 (November 1985): 2103.

29. Bone fractures are possible during the convulsions, though the use of muscle relaxants during the treatment reduces this possibility. Death is a remote possibility by medical standards: approximately 1 patient per 1,000 dies because of cardiac or brain injury during the procedure. Patients with known cardiac problems are watched more carefully or possibly excluded from the procedure.

30. In fact, the patient described lost her memory to the point of having to give up her position as a professional economist.

31. Because of the uncertain risks attending ECT, patients may come to believe their own treatment will "beat the odds." Physicians view this positive attitude as beneficial to the ultimate success of the treatment.

32. See, e.g., California Welfare & Institutions Code § 5326.75 (West 1984) (a psychiatrist or neurologist other than the patient's treating physician must verify that the patient has the capacity to give, and has given, a written informed consent). See also, Note, "Regulation of Electroconvulsive Therapy," *Michigan Law Review* 75, no. 2 (1976): 363.

33. *Blue Shield of Virginia* v. *McCready,* 457 U.S. 465, 102 S. Ct. 2540 (1982).

34. *American Medical Association* v. *Federal Trade Commission,* 638 F. 2d 443 (2d Cir. 1980).

35. *Wilk* v. *American Medical Association,* 635 F. 2d 1295 (7th Cir. 1981).

Chapter 4: Caring for the Critically Ill

1. *In re Haymer,* 450 N.E. 2d 940, 115 Ill. App. 3d 349 (Ill. App. Ct. 1983).

2. In fact, Alex's heart did stop before the case went to trial, and the ventilation system was then disconnected. The case was not declared moot, however, because a judicial declaration accepting "brain death" as a valid definition of death was being sought. The Illinois state legislature does not have a statutory definition of death, although, for the purposes of the Uniform Anatomical Gift Act, the Illinois General Assembly has stated that death means the irreversible cessation of total brain function (Ill. Rev. Stat. chapter 110 1/2, § 302(b) (1981)).

3. Surrounding circumstances in this case raise some suspicion regarding the parents' motives in seeking to maintain use of the life-support system. An affidavit from the medical examiner warned that continued use of the

ventilator system after brain death could lead to tissue deterioration and destabilization, making a determination of the precise cause of death impossible. Were the parents actually seeking to hide a case of child abuse? Was this an underlying assumption of the court, shedding important light on the stark lack of parental consideration in the written opinion? It is also worth noting that some defendants in criminal trials have claimed that the turning off of a life-support system was an intervening cause of the victim's death (e.g., *People* v. *Mitchell,* 132 Cal. App. 3d 389, 183 Cal. Rptr. 166 (1982)).

4. The physicians would have to explain that, despite the fact that the infant was clearly breathing and its heart was functioning, "brain death" was nonetheless a more realistic diagnosis. In light of the growing need for organ transplantations, they would explain, the medical community and many state legislatures felt that the brain-death definition allowed noncognitive patients, often through their families, to confer a substantial health benefit on others who would otherwise die. Such an explanation at least clarifies the social purpose behind the brain-death definition and the necessity of declaring the death as soon as one is certain, so that the organs are still capable of being transplanted. Parents may feel better about the tragic situation knowing that other children will be helped. Some parents may still refuse to accept this social rationale, but regardless of the parents' response, such explanations are vital to confrontations between medical professionals and parents. If the conversation ultimately fails to shift the objecting parents' view, the hospital and physicians could still turn off the ventilator system without parental consent, risking a lawsuit but establishing a set and articulated policy that the court would probably accept. (Note, however, that physicians still would not be able to take a "brain dead" infant's organs for transplantation without parental consent.)

5. In addition, the parents might ask the local prosecutor to begin a criminal case against the physicians, but the crucial issue would still be whether or not the brain-death standard is appropriate. If there was a suspicion of parental battering, the prosecutor would still proceed with the case against the parents when it was clear that the child was critically ill and possibly dead upon arrival at the hospital.

6. *In re Storar,* 52 N.Y. 2d 363, 420 N.E. 2d 64 (1981).

7. When the physicians at the residential facilities first noticed blood in Storar's urine, the mother refused permission to conduct diagnostic tests. After conversations with the center's staff, she agreed to the test and later to radiation treatment, which led to a remission. Within half a year the physicians again noticed blood in Storar's urine, and diagnostic tests subsequently determined that the cancer was terminal. Two months after this diagnosis, the physicians asked the mother for permission to do blood transfusions. She objected but withdrew her objection the next day. Her son received blood transfusions whenever his physicians thought they were

needed. A month later, however, she requested that the transfusions be discontinued, at which point the litigation ensued.

8. 52 N.Y. 2d 363, 388 (Jones, J., dissenting).

9. Notice that under the position proposed here the prosecutor would not have standing to bring a suit since his role is to review actions for possible criminal liability after the fact. We have started to modify this role of the prosecutor in a number of suits involving health care decision-making without specifically discussing the modification. As will be demonstrated later, there are good reasons for maintaining the role of the prosecutor as the reviewer of actions because of the potentially beneficial function of criminal law. A prosecutor convinced that the courts have a limited role would ideally be able to seek the court's permission not to participate in these cases. The legal environment in which the New York court decided Brother Fox's and John Storar's cases did not allow the prosecutor to decline from participating.

10. See *In re Dinnerstein,* 6 Mass. App. Ct. 466, 380 N.E. 2d 134 (1978) and *Saikewicz,* 370 N.E. 2d 417 (1977).

11. *In re Quinlan,* 70 N.J. 355 A. 2d 647 (1976).

12. See New York Public Health Law § 2960–78 (West Supp. 1988).

13. 486 A. 2d 1209, 98 N.J. 321 (1985).

14. 486 A. 2d 1209, 1217.

15. Id. at 1216. Note here the similarity between her symptoms and those of Mrs. Lake in Burt's book *Taking Care of Strangers: The Rule of Law in Doctor-Patient Relations* (New York: Free Press, 1979). I wonder if the court did not discuss the circumstances of her incompetence because it might have been an implicit criticism of the nephew. Also, the court does not see that it could have made a distinction between the adjudication of incompetency and the decision to place in a nursing home.

16. Whether the nursing home is a place for elderly persons to "live out the rest of their lives" or a place where they are sent to die is an issue underlying much of the court's opinion but never openly discussed.

17. 486 A. 2d at 1218 (emphasis added).

18. Id. at 1216.

19. *In re Conroy,* 188 N.J. Super. 523, 457 A. 2d 1232 (1983).

20. 486 A. 2d at 1218.

21. But the court correctly pointed out that the actions of Conroy indicating an antipathy to doctors are not clear and convincing evidence of what she would want to do under the circumstances as stated.

22. 486 A. 2d at 1227.

23. Id. at 1229.

24. Id. at 1232.

25. Id.

26. Id. at 1232–33.

27. Id. at 1219, n.1.
28. Id. at 1237–38.
29. Id. at 1240.
30. Id. at 1242.
31. Id. at 1242–43.
32. Id. at 1220.
33. Id. at 1248.
34. Burt, *Taking Care of Strangers,* pp. 61–65.
35. 188 N.J. Super. 523, 526.
36. 486 A. 2d at 1238–39, n.8, quoting *N.J.S.A.* 30:13-3a,-3b,-3d, and -3g.
37. Id. at 1224–25.
38. Id. at 1217.
39. Id. at 1237.
40. William F. May, *The Physician's Covenant: Images of the Healer in Medical Ethics* (Philadelphia: Westminster Press, 1983), pp. 63–86.

Chapter 5: Legislative Reform and the Question of Dying

1. California Health & Safety Code § 7185–95 (West Supp. 1986).
2. California Health & Safety Code § 7187(c).
3. Alexander M. Capron and Leon R. Kass, "A Statutory Definition of the Standards for Determining Human Death: An Appraisal and a Proposal," *University of Pennsylvania Law Review* 121, no. 1 (November 1972): 87. The case of Alex Hymer, the child defined as "brain dead," was noted in chapter 4.
4. "Terminal condition" means an incurable condition caused by injury, disease, or illness, which, regardless of the application of life-sustaining procedures, would, within reasonable medical judgment, produce death, and where the application of life-sustaining procedures serves only to postpone the moment of death of the patient (California Health & Safety Code § 7187(f)).
5. Burt defines a silent patient as one who cannot communicate his or her treatment preferences, whether because of coma, mental retardation, or similar disability. See his *Taking Care of Strangers: The Rule of Law in Doctor-Patient Relations* (New York: Free Press, 1979), pp. 144–73.
6. California Health & Safety Code § 7191(c).
7. California Health & Safety Code § 7190.
8. In cases where the patient signs a directive *after* receiving knowledge of his or her terminal condition, the attending physician who refuses to carry out the directive is required to find another physician who will follow the patient's directive (California Health & Safety Code § 7191(b)).
9. California Civil Code §§ 2430–44. The statute makes this recognition

of the family in a negative fashion by providing that if there is a marital dissolution after the signing of the durable power of attorney, the designation is revoked by the marital dissolution without any other act, unless there is a specific provision in the appointment of the durable attorney that states it should survive the marital dissolution (California Civil Code § 2437(e)).

10. California Civil Code § 2435.

11. California Civil Code § 2438(c).

12. See Peter Mudd, "High Ideals and Hard Cases: The Evolution of a Hospice," *Hastings Center Report* 12, no. 2 (April 1982): 11.

13. Arnold S. Trebach, *The Heroin Solution* (New Haven: Yale University Press, 1982). Under the Comprehensive Drug Abuse Prevention and Control Act of 1970, heroin may not be used in the practice of American medicine, although morphine and cocaine may (84 Stat. 1236 (1970)). "Once it is accepted that a person's cancer probably will not be controlled, then the dominant theme of treatment should become comfort, not cure. . . . That is where the hospice and the proper use of analgesic drugs should come into the discussion" (Trebach, *Solution,* p. 33). Heroin is widely used in Great Britain, especially in hospices for the treatment of pain related to terminal cancer.

14. The court mentions that the family signed a written request to remove the life-support system but did not include the entire language of the request, including the release from liability (147 Cal. App. 3d at 1009, 195 Cal. Rptr. 486). The language that is quoted in the text is found in *Medical Staff Monthly,* December 1984, p. 1 (a publication of Horty, Springer & Mattern, P.C., Pittsburgh, Pa.).

15. *People* v. *Barber,* No. A 25 586 at 5 (Los Angeles Mun. Ct. Mar. 9, 1983) (magistrate's findings).

16. Id. at 4. Encephalomalacia is softening of the brain because of degenerative changes in the nervous tissue; anoxia is tissue deterioration because of oxygen deficiency.

17. Id. at 4.

18. Id. at 4.

19. Even though the intermediate appellate court eventually held that indictment—the legal pronouncement that there was sufficient cause to let a jury hear the full evidence—was itself insufficient, the legislature ought to consider legislation to establish when doctors are criminally liable for terminating treatment.

20. *People* v. *Barber,* No. A 025586 (Super. Ct. of Cal. May 5, 1983) (tentative findings).

21. California Health & Safety Code § 7195.

22. *People* v. *Barber,* at 5 (Mun. Ct.). California defines death as the irreversible cessation of circulatory and respiratory functions or entire brain functions, including the brain stem (Uniform Determination of Death Act,

California Health & Safety Code § 7180 (West Supp. 1986)). Thus the courts' preoccupation with whether or not Mr. Herbert's condition was irreversible.

23. *People* v. *Barber,* at 4 (Super. Ct.).

24. *Barber* v. *Superior Court of State of California,* 147 Cal. App. 3d 1006, 1011, 195 Cal. Rptr. 484, 486 (1983) (emphasis added).

25. *Barber* v. *Superior Court,* at 1013–14, 195 Cal. L. Rptr. 484, 488.

26. "Nothing in this chapter shall impair or supersede any legal right or legal responsibility which any person may have to effect the withholding or withdrawal of life-sustaining procedures in any lawful manner" (*Barber* v. *Superior Court,* at 1015, 195 Cal. Rptr. 484, 489 (quoting California Health & Safety Code § 7193)).

27. *Barber* v. *Superior Court,* at 1017–20, 195 Cal. Rptr. 484, 491–92.

28. "If the treating physicians have determined that continued use of a respirator is useless, then they may decide to discontinue it without fear of civil or criminal liability" (*Barber* v. *Superior Court,* at 1017, 195 Cal. Rptr. 484, 491 (quoting Dennis Horan, "Euthanasia and Brain Death: Ethical and Legal Considerations," *Annals N.Y. Acad. Sci.* 315 (1978): 363, 367)).

29. Perhaps because the California court was intent on granting total immunity from criminal prosecution, it failed to consider whether the facts could have been construed to include the "lesser included offense" of manslaughter. In modern times, we have developed the concept of vehicular homicide, for instance, which has been used when persons who are driving while intoxicated kill others in an accident. Normally, the killing of persons in an automobile accident is a matter for civil liability, but we recognize our need for the criminal law to provide background legal and moral sanction in an activity that is inherently dangerous. See, e.g., California Penal Code § 192 (West Supp. 1986).

30. The New York Legislature recently passed a statute that dealt specifically with the issue of orders not to resuscitate. The legislation allows a person to indicate in advance his or her wishes regarding resuscitation or to appoint someone else to exercise the right to decline resuscitation in the event of incompetency. See New York Public Health Law §§ 2960–78 (West Supp. 1988), effective April 1988. The statute is both consistent and inconsistent with the approach suggested here. It is consistent with my proposed approach in that it specifically instructs the hospital to establish a mechanism for resolving disputes about resuscitation, implicitly recognizing the social control functions of hospitals as organizations. It is inconsistent by developing an elaborate procedure to deal with the utilization of one piece of medical technology.

31. See William F. May, *The Physician's Covenant: Images of the Healer in Medical Ethics* (Philadelphia: Westminster Press, 1983), pp. 169–92. May's final chapter, "Covenanted Institutions," deals with the problem of medical ethics within the context of the modern hospital.

Chapter 6: Caring for Children

1. *Parham* v. *J. R.,* 442 U.S. 584, 598, 99 S. Ct. 2493, 2502 (1979).

2. The notion of a "voluntary" commitment to a state mental hospital sounds not only like a legal fiction but some type of legal joke. It is hard to imagine anyone, not to mention a child, assenting to commitment, given the conditions of most of these institutions.

3. *In re Gault,* 387 U.S. 1, 87 S. Ct. 1428 (1966).

4. Before the state can deprive an individual of his or her "liberty," it must use a certain type of process which, at minimum, requires notice and an opportunity to contest the facts, as alleged by the state official seeking to incarcerate, in front of a "neutral fact finder." Under this theory, the commitment of a child to a state mental hospital involves a deprivation of the child's liberty by the state officials which thus requires a hearing.

5. 442 U.S. at 597.

6. Some of the cases presented to law involved such questions as whether the child of a Jehovah's Witness should have a blood transfusion during an operation. While these cases involved issues of religious beliefs that were clearly in conflict with the prevailing practice of modern medicine, they did not necessarily represent a total lack of faith in modern medicine. More recently, parents are refusing conventional treatment for their children out of vague but apparently strongly held convictions that reject many of the underlying spiritual and biological assumptions of modern medicine. Nowhere is this more dramatically demonstrated than in instances where parents refuse conventional treatment for cancer and seek alternative treatments.

7. *Custody of a Minor,* 379 N.E. 2d 1053 (1978).

8. Joseph Goldstein, "Medical Care for the Child at Risk: On State Supervision of Parental Autonomy," *Yale Law Journal* 86 (1977): 645, 651.

9. As a matter of fact, the specialist would argue that Chad Green's leukemia was one of the few forms of cancer for which there is a "cure" (379 N.E. 2d 1053).

10. Robert A. Burt, *Taking Care of Strangers: The Rule of Law in Doctor–Patient Relations* (New York: Free Press, 1979), ch. 5 passim.

11. *Hart* v. *Brown,* 29 Conn. Sup. 368 (1972).

12. When asked to donate a kidney, the donor might be expected to experience some ambivalence, but the social pressure to give the kidney does not appear inappropriate if we assume that individuals are connected to one another by complex emotional and psychological bonds. In an ordinary case, no one would think to ask the court for a declaration of the donor's right to donate. We have thus accepted without question the idea that it is "right" to ask some persons to give kidneys so that others may live.

13. I say the hospital and the physicians were seeking legal validation of the experiment because it is difficult to understand what legal risks they

were taking *if the facts are as they were alleged to be.* The one most obvious risk is that the donor child might, as an adult, take the position that the parents were not entitled to consent, making the surgeons liable in damages. In a society that accepts "donation" of human organs as the proper way of obtaining them (having rejected the idea of purchasing human organs), it is hard to imagine how any such lawsuit might succeed. Even at the technical level, the parent would have the authority to consent to the use of the twin in a medical experiment where there were risks, so the lack of direct therapeutic benefit is not a legal basis for the lawsuit.

14. 29 Conn. Sup. at 375.

15. We can imagine a situation where there is a conflict: for example, where the physician recommends the transplantation but the parent (or parents) refuses to assent. Were the physician to bring a lawsuit on the theory that performing the transplant was required by "legal and moral" duty, a court should even here decline to intervene. The physician would be merely trying to impose a personal concept of "health" and thus personal professional values on the parents. Law should reject the tendency to assume that "health" is essentially an objective phenomenon.

16. *Roe* v. *Wade,* 410 U.S. 113, 93 S. Ct. 705 (1973).

17. *Bellotti* v. *Baird (Bellotti II),* 443 U.S. 662, 99 S. Ct. 3035 (1979).

18. *H.L.* v. *Matheson,* 450 U.S. 398, 101 S. Ct. 1164 (1981).

19. In fact, the laws making abortions illegal only originated, for the most part, in the last half of the nineteenth century. Medical abortions were commonly administered even in the Greek times, as well as in the Roman era. (*Roe* v. *Wade,* 410 U.S. at 130.)

20. 410 U.S. 113 (1973).

21. *In re Phillip B.,* 92 Ca. App. 3d 796, 156 Cal. Rptr. 48 (1979).

The unpublished court opinions are reproduced in Walter Wadlington, Charles H. Whitbread, and Samuel M. Davis, *Cases and Materials on Children in the Legal System* (Mineola, N.Y.: Foundation Press, 1983), pp. 921–23.

22. This action is significant because there are instances where parents do, in fact, give up all legal rights to their mentally retarded children who are institutionalized. See 442 U.S. at 617.

23. Phillip's parents sued *Newsweek* for libel in the magazine's coverage of the case. As part of the settlement the parents, Warren M. and Patricia Becker, were allowed to express their views in a "My Turn" column in *Newsweek,* 30 May 1983. In "Mourning the Loss of a Son," the Beckers describe the proceedings in which they lost custody of their child, Phillip, to Herbert and Pat Heath, who had worked with Phillip in the care facility (*New York Times,* 12 July 1983, p. 14).

24. Rita Swan, "Faith Healing, Christian Science, and the Medical Care of Children," *New England Journal of Medicine* 309, no. 26 (December 1983): 1639–41.

Chapter 7: The Path Toward Caring and Justice

1. See Robert E. Keeton, "Compensation for Medical Accidents," *University of Pennsylvania Law Review* 121 (1973): 590, 591–600.

2. *New York Times,* 4 April 1986, p. 1.

3. In addition, the contingent fee system by which plaintiff lawyers are paid in most malpractice suits operates to encourage settlement, since the lawyer has financed the lawsuit up to that point, sometimes over a period of years, and needs to recover his costs.

4. *New York Times,* 12 February 1985, p. 1.

5. McKinney's Session Laws of New York, Chapter 294, 208th Session, 1985 (West 1986).

6. *In the Matter of Baby "M,"* 109 N.J. 396, 537 A. 2d 1227 (1988).

7. See Cornell University, *A Study of the Post-Graduate Activities of the Class of 1987, Cornell University* (Ithaca, N.Y.: Cornell University, 1988). This recent survey of Cornell graduates found (p. 3) that 26 percent of the 1987 graduating class will go on to graduate or professional school.

8. See Donald A. Schön, *The Reflective Practitioner: How Professionals Think in Action* (New York: Basic Books, 1983); id., *Educating the Reflective Practitioner: Toward a New Design for Teaching and Learning in the Professions* (San Francisco: Jossey-Bass Publishers, 1987). See also Alfred Aman, "Studying Music, Learning Law: A Musical Perspective on Clinical Legal Education," *Cornell Law Forum* 13 (February 1987): 8.

9. See generally William F. May, *The Physician's Covenant: Images of the Healer in Medical Ethics* (Philadelphia: Westminster Press, 1983). May's notion of the professional relationship in terms of a covenant rather than contract could be infused in clinical and interdisciplinary teaching in law schools.

10. See Larry Palmer, "Research on Human Subjects as a Paradigm in Teaching," *Law, Medicine and Health Care* 16, no. 2/3 (Summer/Fall 1988).

11. Two recent examinations are Larry Churchill, *Rationing Health Care in America* (Notre Dame, Ind.: University of Notre Dame Press, 1987), and Charles J. Dougherty, *American Health Care: Realities, Rights, and Reforms* (New York: Oxford University Press, 1988). For reasons that will become apparent, I believe Churchill's approach to these problems is more compatible with the approach suggested here.

12. Dougherty, *American Health Care,* pp. 116–20.

13. See chapter 1 for discussion of entitlements.

14. *Sidaway* v. *Board of Governors of the Bethlem Royal Hospital,* 2 W.L.R. 480 (1985).

15. Id.

16. Robert Schwartz and Andrew Grubb, "Why Britain Cannot Afford Informed Consent," *Hastings Center Report* 15, no. 4 (August 1985): 19.

17. *Washington Post,* 2 July 1988, p. 49.

18. Note "Rethinking Medical Malpractice Law in Light of Medical Cost-Cutting," *Harvard Law Review* 98 (1985): 1004.

19. See Sander Gilman, *Disease and Representation: Images of Illness from Madness to AIDS* (Ithaca, N.Y.: Cornell University Press, 1988), pp. 245–72.

Index

Abortion: genetic health issues involving, 27–34; legal imposition of, as therapeutic alternative, 31; for minors, 109, 117–120; public ambivalence about, 9; right to, 30, 144n42
Abortion clinics, 120
Acquired Immune Deficiency Syndrome (AIDS), 17, 137
Administrative agencies, and social obligations of physicians, 62–63, 70–71
Adolescent, rights of, 110
AHA. *See* American Hospital Association (AHA)
AIDS. *See* Acquired Immune Deficiency Syndrome (AIDS)
Allopathic medicine, 150n12
AMA. *See* American Medical Association (AMA)
American Association for Cancer Research, 42
American Hospital Association (AHA), 69
American Medical Association (AMA): Principles of Medical Ethics, 64; structure of health care delivery and, 69–70
Amniocentesis, 28
Artificial heart program, 36–38
Artistry, professionalism as, 133–134

Baby Jane Doe case, 53, 62–63
Baby M case, 131, 143n33

Bacon, Francis, 90–91
Battered child syndrome, 58–62, 75–76, 156n5
Becker v. *Schwartz*, 28–33
Berman v. *Allan*, 29–33
Biomedical advances: communal values and, 131; concepts of health and, 52; death with dignity and, 87–88; expectations for physicians and, 127–128; institutional approach and, 37–38; institutional review boards and, 37–38; liability rules and, 26; medical misadventure and, 127; role of physician and, 63, 126; scientific approach to medicine and, 8–9
Biomedical research: medical role in social control and, 44–48; prestige and, 149n10; role of hospitals in, 40–44
Blood transfer, 17, 142n18
Blood transfusion, as treatment, 78–83
Brain death, 20–21, 73, 95, 100, 102–103, 141n16, 160n4, 160n5
Burger, Warren, 112
Burt, Robert, 96, 115

California: "natural" death legislation in, 94–104, 163n22
Caretaking institutions: compelling treatment in, 53–55; deinstitutionalization and, 56–57; institution of medicine in, 39–40; as jurisdiction for legal conflicts, 39–40, 48–57; medical

DATE DUE

OC25 '96			
NO25 '96			